OUT OF THE BOX & OVER THE BARRIERS

Community-Driven Strategies
for Addressing the Uninsured

**Vondie Moore Woodbury
Donna Strugar-Fritsch
Pamela Paul Shaheen**

ISBN: 1-4033-8472-X (electronic)
ISBN: 1-4033-8473-8 (softcover)

Library of Congress Control Number: 2002095141

This book is printed on acid free paper.

Printed in the United States of America
Bloomington, IN

1st Books – rev. 10/17/02

This manual is a joint effort of the
Center for Advancing Community Health and the
Muskegon Community Health Project.
It is based on our experiences in creating *Access Health©*, a
program to provide health care coverage to the working
uninsured in Muskegon County, Michigan.

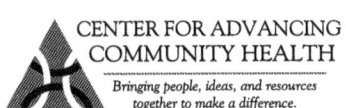 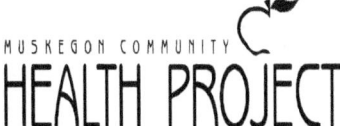

Funding of the Muskegon Community Health Project and
funds to develop this book were generously provided by the
W.K. Kellogg Foundation.

We would like to acknowledge the following people for their
contributions to this manual:

Gary Packingham for creative influence

Sally Bancroft for graphic design

Eileen Ellis, Health Management Associates,
for technical assistance

CONTENTS

Chapter.....1

Why this manual?

- Introduction
- Using the Manual

INTRODUCTION

As the United States enters the 21st century, more than 44 million Americans do not have health insurance. In the "best" states, 9 percent of residents have no insurance; in the worst, 28 percent lack coverage.

The good news is that for the first time since monitoring began, the proportion of residents without health insurance has dropped. The overall uninsured rate dropped from 16.3 percent in 1998 to 15.5 percent in 1999. Credit for this drop is given to the expansion of programs like the federal CHIP (Children's' Health Insurance Program) and to a robust economy in which people have more access to employer-sponsored health benefits.

In spite of this improvement, lack of health insurance remains a very real and significant issue for many individuals within our communities. Minority populations and individuals who work in low-wage occupations, such as those in the retail and service sectors, continue to have far less health insurance coverage than average. Children also continue to fall short in terms of coverage, in spite of major government-sponsored initiatives. It also is important to recognize that, while U.S. residents as a whole are reaping the benefits of a prosperous economy as the new millennium begins, employer-sponsored health insurance benefits remain dependent upon the strength of our economy. When an economic downturn comes, decreasing levels of health insurance are almost certain to follow. For some employers, providing health insurance to their employees and their families may be a short-term phenomenon, lasting only as long as the pressure to recruit and retain a skilled workforce during a time of record low unemployment rates.

Another recognized phenomenon is the growing category of people who are considered "under-insured." By definition, under-insurance exists when the health coverage a person has is so limited and the resources that person has are so few that he or she is unable to seek a doctor's care except in instances of extreme illness or emergency. As alarming as it is, health economists see this trend increasing significantly over the next decade. As pharmacy costs, health insurance premiums, and other employer-related health insurance costs increase, employers are shifting the burden to the employees. Employees are facing ever-increasing health insurance copays and deductibles, reduced benefits,

As alarming as it is, health economists see trends in uninsurance and under-insurance rates rising significantly over the next decade.

lifetime limits, and higher out-of-pocket expenses. Experts say this trend toward reduced insurance coverage and increased out-of-pocket expenses will create a growing sector of under-insured residents in virtually all communities, a situation that will impact the entire whole local health system.

"Health care access" is a broad issue with many facets. Access to health care services encompasses issues of insurance and health care coverage, but also other issues that are beyond the scope of this manual. Among these issues are:

- Maldistribution of doctors, dentists, and other health care service providers;
- Maldistribution of health care facilities, such as emergency rooms, clinics, and hospitals;
- Provider acceptance of Medicaid and other forms of coverage;
- Racial, ethnic, and cultural disparities in care;
- Transportation and accessibility barriers; and
- Capacity versus demand.

Although we recognize the vital importance of each of these issues, in this manual we limit our focus to methods to create *access to health care services* and/or *access to payment for insurance or coverage.*

Communities throughout the United States are testing innovative strategies to provide health care to the uninsured and to expand coverage for those individuals who are under-insured. Some have achieved success through unique methods of insurance or other forms of coverage. Others have found means to provide access to health care services. There are successful examples, but no one model is directly applicable to other communities. Subtle and not-so-subtle differences between communities make it seem like each group of reformers must start from scratch in designing their problem solving approaches, a testimony to the rock-solid premise that all health care is local.

In Muskegon County, Michigan, we created *Access Health©,* a health coverage program sold to small businesses to extend health care coverage to the working uninsured. Our model is very tailored to our community, and the path to *Access Health©* was long, but ultimately productive.

Looking back, we found that much of what we went through could have been easier and faster if we had the right kind of resources to engage the members of our community in our efforts. While there are many resources available on the topic of engaging communities to address health issues, and consultants abound, most of those resources and consultant services are provider-driven, meaning they are targeted at hospitals, health systems, or local public health departments. We found that these provider-driven models of community engagement and health care reform did not adequately address the diverse points of view that exist among those who purchase health care services and those who provide them. Also, very few models focus on providing financial coverage for care.

We believe the lessons we learned in Muskegon County apply to any community seeking solutions for its uninsured and under-insured residents. They are especially applicable to small- and medium-sized communities. We created this manual as a resource to smooth the way for communities like ours who need funding coverage or services for the uninsured – for communities that seek effective solutions that are supported by business, local government, and the health care sector. If that describes your community, read on...

We created this manual as a resource for communities that want effective, locally-driven solutions for the uninsured. It is especially applicable to medium-sized and small communities.

USING THE MANUAL

This manual presents a framework from which to study and address the issues of health care for the uninsured and under-insured. It provides both an overview of the steps necessary to produce viable local solutions and case study examples. The manual is divided into chapters, and includes references, appendices, and an epilogue in which we describe the impact of *Access Health©* in our community.

A note: the manual is written as though your community is just getting started, and has no organized efforts underway. For some of you, that won't be true. Your community may already have grassroots activities in progress, or a health council involving the local health power brokers, or other efforts. The manual can still be very useful, especially in suggesting ways to integrate existing activities and structures with some new ones that will engage other stakeholders, and give you a community-wide strategy. We encourage you to keep an open mind as you read, and don't feel like we are telling you to undo what already exists. Look for ways to augment and improve your process, which will result in stronger, more sustainable interventions.

CHAPTER SUMMARIES

Chapter One: Why This Manual?

This chapter provides an overview to the issue of coverage for health care, trends, the role of community in addressing its unique health care circumstances, and an overview of the manual.

Chapter Two: Get Ready

This chapter has two purposes:

- It explains and justifies the legitimate role of communities in owning and addressing issues of access to health care.

- It guides you through a study of the characteristics and the motivations of the many health care stakeholders in your community. In this process, the participants will develop a common language and commonly held general information about the uninsured and become familiar with one another's diverse but legitimate points of view and self-interest. This knowledge is a crucial underpinning of a successful community effort.

Chapter Three: Groundwork to Stimulate Local Political Will for Change

This chapter describes the need to generate political will for changing the status quo regarding the uninsured. It also provides steps to generate political will, including:

- studying the community's unique circumstances with respect to its health care, and

- "firing up" the community's interest in addressing the situation.

Chapter Four: Build and Use a Legitimate Community-Driven Engine for Change

This chapter outlines a process for formalizing local structures for both governance and action planning, so that together they will produce and support "real" community-driven strategies for change. It details the objectives and strategies of a governing body and of community-based work teams, as well as methods for integrating the two.

Chapter Five: Study Your Uninsured and Under-Insured

Many communities (or stakeholder groups within the community) believe that they already understand "the uninsured." This chapter outlines questions and issues your community must explore in detail in order to thoroughly understand your local situation and what must be done to address it.

Chapter Six: Planning for Change

This chapter presents a framework you can use to explore an array of methods that other communities have used to provide coverage for health care for the uninsured. It also helps your community identify its needs and circumstances, depending upon a wide variety of factors, thus enabling your community to narrow the focus of solutions you might consider.

In each chapter, we will provide Action Tips on how to locally manage certain issues that arise at every step. These include:
- Objectives
- Organizing
- Who pays?
- Decision making
- Record keeping
- Strategies for conveners
- Hazards and traps
- Additional resources

It is important to mention that you won't find a prescribed answer for your community in this chapter or anywhere else in this manual; selecting your community's individual solution is your community's responsibility. Instead, you will learn about the many ways you can help address the health coverage needs of your residents who are living without insurance, and a method to guide your community to a strategy that fits its particular circumstances. This chapter also will prepare you to deal with details of governance, finance, risk, and others as they apply to your situation.

Chapter Seven: Implementation

This chapter prepares you for life *after* you have created a locally driven, locally supported method of caring for the uninsured. This chapter is based upon our direct experiences with *Access Health©*. In it, we share what we would have done differently to more accurately anticipate and prevent problems, market the program, engage the media, design data collection and reporting systems, and address other very important issues. This chapter will equip you with information we wish we had thought through more thoroughly before jumping into the water.

Epilogue

Here we describe the history of *Access Health©* and what it has done for the working uninsured in Muskegon County.

Chapter.....2

Get Ready............

- The Role of Community in Providing Care for Its Uninsured

- Access to Health Care: Many Perspectives

- Introduce the Stakeholders: I'm OK, You May Not Be

THE ROLE OF COMMUNITY IN PROVIDING CARE FOR ITS UNINSURED

The dichotomy facing communities as they address health care access issues is that the arena of "health" is a complex combination of financial and social interests, issues, and systems. These elements are so intertwined at the local level that to deal with one without considering the others is to ask for failure.

A community's quality of life, viability of its businesses, and integrity of its health system are interwoven. The population's health status impacts the local workforce, student performance, welfare and other safety nets, and health care costs. The health system impacts business costs and public services. Uninsured populations impact health systems, businesses, schools, public programs, and providers.

There is a legitimate role for a community to take charge of its own uninsured population and to weave federal, state, and local strategies into a tapestry that covers its unique population.

The maxim "all health is local" is as true today as it always has been. Much of our health system is determined by federal and state governments, and many health services are delivered through organizations owned and governed outside of the community. However, we still *receive* our health care in our neighborhoods and local communities, and each community is different from the next in its citizens, values, and organizations.

Federal and state government-designed interventions to address the uninsured focus largely on either tax cuts or entitlement programs. For instance, businesses are offered tax cuts as incentives to offer health insurance benefits, or eligibility requirements for Medicaid are revised, and new entitlements, like the CHIP program, are created. Other federal initiatives address maldistribution issues — Federally Qualified Health Centers receive special levels of reimbursement to allow higher payment to doctors who practice in under-served urban or rural locations; medical education loan forgiveness programs place doctors and nurses in underserved areas.

These externally imposed strategies address either the business of health or its social side, not both. As such, they may alter a community's uninsured programs, but they fall far short of comprehensive solutions that satisfy the financial and social concerns of a unique community. Thus, a community can play a legitimate productive role by taking charge of its own uninsured population and weaving federal, state, and local strategies into a tapestry that covers its unique population.

If you aren't yet convinced of the community's rightful place in crafting local solutions to access to health care, consider that:

- More than 1,600 communities applied for $20 million in grants offered by the U.S. government's Health Resources and Services Administration in 1999.
- Foundations and the federal government are making large amounts of money available to communities to fund innovative local strategies to address the uninsured.

Funds have been made available because there is evidence that communities are capable of addressing this complex issue. It is both the role and the privilege of each community to assert its values and determine how to address the complex issue of people lacking health insurance coverage within its unique array of local circumstances and stakeholders. It is the task of each community to integrate the social and business sides of the uninsured through local partnerships and creative local strategies. It is the role of each community to own and tend the health of its population, and to invest in its health care system. Indeed, only the individual community can do the job in the way that it needs to be done.

When we speak of *the uninsured,* we are speaking of people who do not have access to insurance coverage for health services. The individuals who make up "the uninsured" do not have health insurance from entitlement programs, self-purchased policies, or employer-sponsored benefits.

Providing insurance for health care addresses one element of access for these individuals – it provides financial coverage. However, there may be other barriers to obtaining health care. For instance, a community resident may have dental insurance, but can find no local dentist who accepts that insurance. That resident has coverage, but not access to care.

Your community must thoroughly look at *access to health care services* and *access to payment for insurance or coverage.* But, your community also will need to address other barriers to health care access.

ACCESS TO HEALTH CARE: SO MANY PERSPECTIVES

It is crucial that the stakeholders in a community accept one another's diverse points of view about the uninsured as legitimate.

When it comes to local health issues, financial and social stakeholders abound. And many of the resources on collaborative processes will show you ways to manage diversity, be inclusive, and build trust. (References to several of these books, organizations, and websites are included in the manual.) But in Muskegon, we found that before our stakeholders could engage in useful dialogue, they first needed to hear and understand each other's points of view. After they understood each other's stake, they were able to work together to develop solutions that honored both the financial and social points of view held by all the stakeholders in our community.

The process to address the uninsured can become very contentious; all of the stakeholders feel passionately about "the uninsured," though for very different reasons. It is vitally important to understand who has a vested interest, why, and what that interest is. It is even more crucial to accept the various points of view as legitimate. It is important to acquaint the stakeholders with one another to reduce intimidation among them. Traditionally, health care discussions have been the domain of the hospitals, doctors, and employers' human resources departments. Other stakeholders may be intimidated by these "experts."

At the risk of making sweeping generalizations about the stakeholders, let us do just that. Here, based upon our experience, are brief summaries of the categories of stakeholders, as well as broad descriptions of how they generally perceive the issue of uninsured populations. We present them alphabetically, and remind you that while each is important, the uninsured and under-insured themselves are the community's central consideration. Your job will be to explore these perspectives in more detail in your community.

Chamber of Commerce

· The local Chamber of Commerce represents local small businesses and offers services and products to its members, such as group purchasing and life insurance.

- Many Chambers also sell employee health insurance to their members. As such, your Chamber may perceive a local alternative to providing employee health insurance (one strategy for addressing the uninsured) as competition for its insurance products.

Community Mental Health Providers

- Local Community Mental Health Boards (CMHBs) are charged with providing mental health services to the persistently and chronically mentally ill and to persons with developmental disabilities.

- Many communities struggle with the coordination of medical service to the CMHB population. Funding and systems are very fragmented.

- Coordination of care challenges are more difficult when clients are "dually diagnosed" with mental illness or a developmental disability *and* a chronic medical or substance abuse problem.

- Portions of a local indigent population often weave in and out of a CMHB's caseload.

Community Philanthropy

- Community philanthropists include agencies like United Way, community foundations, and local corporate and family foundations or private donors.

- They often are asked to fund gaps in local systems, and they are likely to be interested in exploring viable local strategies that would effectively close the gaps instead of temporarily plugging them over and over.

County or Local Government

- Elected officials have some degree of responsibility to provide medical services to those without access to care.

- The degree of responsibility varies by statute and also by practice. For instance, some county governments operate public hospitals or long term care facilities; others do not. Some are actively involved in funding clinics or services; others budget only minimally for such expenses.

The stakeholder descriptions we share are deliberately general and are provided just to get you started on a path to discovering the stakeholder point of view in your community.

- There may be significant (and historic) turf issues between city or township, county, and state government with respect to responsibility for the uninsured.

- If county or local officials have not been involved in health services in the past, they are likely to have a steep learning curve.

Economic Development

- Economic development organizations are usually in the public sector and exist to attract business to the community. The quality of life in the community is a vital element in their ability to compete for new business and industry.

- The "competitors" for new business and industry are no longer just neighboring communities in your state or even other states. International competition within a global economy is an increasing reality.

- Potential business and industry place a high value on health care quality, competitive costs, and a continuum of health services that meet employee needs. The local level of the uninsured may impact all of these.

- Potential business and industry also consider the health of the community's residents. A healthy, robust workforce is more attractive than a workforce drawn from a community with high levels of chronic disease and substance abuse.

Faith-Based Community

- People turn to their spiritual leaders and support systems in times of sickness and financial hardship. That means the faith-based community may be the first to know about health care problems in the community. This sector has a clear picture of the way local health systems and issues play out in the lives of real people.

- Faith communities across the country are developing new social service networks through health screening programs for their worshippers, parish nurse programs, healing ministries, and other organized efforts.

- Some organized religions actively view health as an issue of social justice; others view health on a more individual basis, as it impacts a person or a group of people.

Farmers

- Farmers will have many of the same health insurance issues as small businesses, but there also are access and health status issues that are unique to farming families.

- If your community includes farmers, you will want to consider them as a unique constituency.

Federally Qualified Health Centers (FQHCs)

- Federally Qualified Health Centers (FQHCs) receive special levels of reimbursement from the federal government for delivering primary care to otherwise underserved populations.

- This reimbursement level helps recruit doctors and deliver services customized to the unique population.

- FQHCs are located in rural or center-city urban areas, and their service population may include migrants.

- FQHCs are already well acquainted with the indigent population.

- In some areas, an FQHC can lose its designation, and therefore its preferential reimbursement, if the level of uninsured drops low enough to no longer qualify the area as underserved.

Hospitals

- Historically, most hospitals began with charitable missions, often faith-based ones. Recently, all have adopted business models and methods. Many have become part of, or have evolved into, larger health systems. The components of systems vary widely.

- Hospitals usually provide uncompensated care through emergency rooms and other inpatient services to people without insurance. That means they receive no payment for these services.

- Hospitals are required by federal law to stabilize anyone appearing in the emergency room.

- All hospitals are experiencing financial strains based upon the recent federal Balanced Budget Amendment, which significantly reduced Medicare payments.

- Depending upon the state, hospitals may have ongoing funding struggles with Medicaid.

- A hospital's level of uncompensated care depends upon many factors, including:
  - The presence of other hospitals;
  - The hospital's historic and geographic position within the community;
  - The local alternatives to the hospital's ER and inpatient care;
  - The hospital's mission, including profit versus not-for-profit status; and
  - The mix of services provided by the hospital.

- For a variety of reasons, there are often inequities in the level of uncompensated care between hospitals. It is a sensitive topic in most communities.

- Hospitals tend to be guarded in collaboration with other hospitals; historic and current competition is often a factor, either explicitly or otherwise.

Immigrant Populations

- Communities vary widely in the presence and fluctuation of immigrant populations. U.S. immigration policy also changes regularly, and can result in unanticipated immigration of new ethnic groups for which a community may not be prepared.

- Each immigrant population has its own cultural issues associated with health and seeking care, which must be respected and addressed in any health care strategy.

- Different health care access issues are associated with documented and undocumented alien residents, and require highly tailored approaches.

Indigent Residents

- This population is very different from the working uninsured in terms of their health care and social service needs.

- The indigent do not meet eligibility criteria for Medicaid or most other government-sponsored programs. They are primarily adult males, ages 19 — 64, who fall between the cracks of Medicaid and Medicare. Some indigent residents may also be women without children, in the same age group.

- Indigent residents need a safety net, wrap-around services, and strong local case management.

- Often these residents receive health care only through emergency rooms and after a medical condition has advanced.

- Effective preventive or primary care for the indigent requires tailored outreach and case management, coupled with an understanding of the population and its needs.

Large Business

- It is important to understand the degree to which a large employer is vested in the local issue of the uninsured.

- Large employers are often based outside the community, and the realities of mergers and acquisitions often reduce their interest in local issues.

- Large businesses vary widely in offering health insurance to some, all, or most employees, depending upon eligibility policies, mandatory waiting periods, unionization, and other factors.

Local Public Health

- Local Public Health Departments (LPHDs) vary widely within states and across the country in their size and sophistication.

- All are charged with responsibility for ensuring health services to at-risk and underserved populations.

- Some LPHDs are direct service providers; others are not.

- In those areas where LPHDs are direct service providers, they are often perceived to compete with private sector providers.

- LPHDs have expertise in cultural competency with diverse populations, such as the homeless, migrants, and ethnic minorities.

- LPHDs usually maintain large amounts of local community health data.

- An LPHD may have initiated a community health status assessment program or process. It may also feel entitled to be the convener or leader of such a process.

- Your LPHD may cover a number of communities. It is labor-intensive and difficult for an LPHD to engage in community processes in multiple communities.

Managed Care Organizations (HMOs, PPOs)

- Generally, Managed Care Organizations (MCOs) view the uninsured as beyond their scope of responsibility, which is limited to caring for "enrollees" or "covered lives" (i.e., people for whom they receive premium payments).

- Regardless, MCOs may be partners in providing care to the uninsured.

- If an MCO has Medicaid beneficiaries as enrollees, it will have strong feelings about the uninsured population, but those will vary with the circumstance. For instance:

  - An MCO experienced with the Medicaid population may have effective outreach activities and a focus on cultural competency.

  - An MCO may also be more or less financially disposed to deal with the uninsured, depending upon Medicaid reimbursement rates and other local reimbursement circumstances.

- An MCO whose enrolled populations are all "commercial" or employer-based will probably have trouble shifting gears to care for enrollees without transportation, or who have had no health care for many years, or who don't "know how" to relate to a primary care physician.

Minority Advocates

- Racial and ethnic minority groups vary widely in their values and norms regarding health care and health insurance coverage. Racial and ethnic values run deep, and some minority groups are distrustful of traditionalnetworks.

- It is critical to include representatives of local minorities (e.g., the Urban League, the National Association for the Advancement of Colored People, local ethnic groups, and faith-based organizations) in community health efforts, both to understand the access issues unique to each minority population and to design strategies that can effectively address those circumstances.

- It is important to bring minority groups into the planning process early, and not to assume that you already know their concerns.

Organized Labor

- In some communities, organized labor sees the lack of health insurance as a force driving the desire to unionize.

- Solving the problem of the working uninsured may be viewed as threatening to labor's objectives.

Physicians

- Physicians tend to view the uninsured "one patient at a time." As such, they tend to lack a systems perspective.

- In general, doctors are frustrated with current trends in payment, autonomy, managed care, and insurance.

- It is extremely difficult to engage physicians in local problem solving networks. Their orientation is to see patients in their offices or hospitals, and time spent in meetings is both a clinical and financial imposition. Where there are physician practice groups, it often is more practical to engage an administrator (if there is one) in your process.

- In most parts of the country, relationships between physicians and hospitals or health systems are tense, or at least wary. There is a transition underway to cooperative working relationships, but it has not yet fully developed.

Retirees

- Retirees are increasingly uninsured, as the gap between retirement age and the age limit for Medicare eligibility grows.

- The Medicare program includes significant deductibles and copays, which create access issues for low-income retirees.

- While retirees from large businesses often receive or purchase supplemental Medigap-type insurance coverage, many retirees do not. Under-insurance is therefore an issue.

- Prescription drug costs are an increasing problem for retirees on fixed incomes, whether or not they have supplemental Medicare insurance.

Safety Net Providers

- Local nonprofits and government-sponsored programs form the safety net in most communities. They provide services for populations like the homeless and substance abusers, and services like food banks, shelters, and counseling practices.

- Safety net providers see their cascloads rise as the levels of uninsurance in a community rise, yet their own operating resources do not rise accordingly.

Small Business

- Small businesses are usually in the retail or service sectors, both of which traditionally provide low-wage jobs.

- Local small businesses may or may not provide employees with health insurance benefits.

- Those who do provide these benefits may feel strongly about those who do not.

- Those who do not provide insurance usually feel that they cannot do so because of high costs.

- More small businesses are currently offering employee health insurance as a tool to recruit and retain employees in a tight labor market.

- Many small businesses have ten or fewer employees.

Sole Proprietors

- The number of these businesses, which consist of one owner/employee, is increasing all over the country.

- Sole proprietors bear unusually high costs for insurance and have few choices, because they often are not eligible for group purchasing arrangements.

- Sole proprietors face especially high burdens if illness or disease interferes with their ability to work.

Under-Insured Residents

- The number of under-insured residents is changing rapidly in many communities. You will need to closely study your local trends in coverage and out-of-pocket expenses.

- Under-insured residents add to the health system's levels of uncompensated care, and you also will need to examine this trend in your community.

- Under-insured people often delay preventive care, diagnostics, and/or treatment because they are unable to pay for their portion of expenses.

Working Uninsured

- Typically, the working uninsured work for small local businesses or work part-time for large businesses. They generally maintain steady employment, but often are paid low or very low wages.

- Often, the working uninsured are referred to as "the working poor." However, they do not identify themselves as "poor," which has pejorative connotations. They view themselves as self-sufficient working citizens and very often do not want government services

- Often, these adults or their children are "entitled," by virtue of eligibility requirements, to Medicaid, food stamps, or other government-sponsored benefits.

- Often, the working uninsured do not want the benefits to which they are entitled and, in fact, have negative views of what they consider to be "handouts" and "welfare."

- Purchasing private health insurance is beyond the financial capabilities of this population.

- The working uninsured may prefer to seek preventive or early care, but often cannot afford it; this conflict often leads to delayed treatment and the associated higher costs.

Armed with these over-generalized "assumptions," your community's task is to go deeper among yourselves to refine your understanding of one another's point of view. How? Read on…

INTRODUCE THE STAKEHOLDERS: I'M OK, YOU MAY NOT BE

The very first step in this long process happens when someone in the community becomes sufficiently concerned about the issue of the uninsured or under-insured to "do something." That first "something" usually is nothing more sophisticated than calling a few like-minded colleagues and kicking around some ideas.

This small, informal group forms the nucleus of your community's process. These folks care about the uninsured, but always from a position of "enlightened self-interest" – the uninsured are a problem for them in some way.

The next step (and the first "official" one) is to draw a larger group together and begin an earnest community dialogue.

ACTION TIPS

The objectives of this step are to:

- Convene a diverse, engaged group that will eventually commit to working together to find a local option for the uninsured.

- Develop a common language and a common understanding of the issues surrounding the uninsured.
- Familiarize the stakeholders with one another's points of view and self-interest.

Organizing: It is crucial that you involve business, people from outside health care, and at least some of your community's minorities, even at this early point.

Your natural inclination will be to convene like-minded colleagues —"friends of the cause." But understand that leadership and participation from only one sector (usually the health care providers) will be perceived as 'suspect" because of self-interest, and will not develop the political will necessary to support change.

Think of the initial group as the skeleton of what will become a community-wide system of checks and balances. Remember that health bridges financial and social realms, and construct your group accordingly.

Your group's leadership can be informal at this point; anyone can serve as chair to convene meetings and set agendas.

Who Pays? The costs for this step include meeting space, refreshments, clerical support, and supplies for mailing and duplication. In general, the cost of the first three meetings can be absorbed by the party with the original idea.

It is usually too early for a group to seek grant funds for this step, although a community foundation or other benefactor may be able to provide seed money to support early discussions.

Decision making is fairly informal at this point, as well, with little need for a formal voting process. At this stage, the dynamics of the group need to support the development of consensus around the importance of the issue, and a formal voting process is not appropriate.

Record keeping is crucial at every step, even now. Records of decisions, assignments, and attendance must be produced, as they may be necessary for conflict resolution later.

A meeting facilitator is a must, but you need not hire an external facilitator. Any neutral, experienced person will do.

Tips for Conveners:

- A meeting facilitator is a must, but you need not hire an external facilitator. Any neutral, experienced person will do.

- Locations that are neutral are preferred, even at this early point. United Ways or other non-health, community-based locations are ideal. Don't meet in a bank board room or other setting that will intimidate community members.

- Get into the habit of leaving titles at the door. Ideally, everyone is addressed by their first and last name.

- Use effective meeting practices: a meaty agenda, prompt beginning and ending times, and refreshments are essential.

- The focus of the initial meetings might be:

  - Discussions of national and state data on the uninsured, and a comparison of national data to what you see in your community;

  - Discussions of the roles of state and federal government in access to health care;

  - Sharing of data or resources from the participants; and

  - Give-and-take discussions of how the participants view the issue of the uninsured.

Hazards and Traps

Consultants are inappropriate at this step, although they themselves may not think so. The community stakeholders need to take ownership of this issue and become a working team with one shared local vision. Deciding on this vision is strictly inside business; resist the urge to look outside for assistance.

Naysayers will attempt to deactivate your group. At this stage, let them express their opinions, which are just as valid as everyone else's.

Haste will tempt you. Avoid the urge to move to solutions or cookbook strategies. Take the time to allow consensus and familiarity to build, as they are the vital ingredients in the important work that follows.

Additional Resources: There are many wonderful references on community process. Here are some of our favorites.

Community-Based Public Health: A Partnership Model, produced by the W.K. Kellogg Foundation and the American Public Health Association, 2000. ISBN # 0-87553-184-9

Collaboration Handbook: Creating, Sustaining and Enjoying the Journey, produced by the Amherst H. Wilder Foundation, 1994. ISBN # 0-940069-03-2

Healthier Communities Action Kit: A Guide for Leaders Embracing Change, produced by the Healthcare Forum Leadership Center, 1993

From the Ground Up! A Workbook on Coalition Building & Community Development, produced by AHEC Community Partners, 1995

The Community Collaboration Manual, produced by the National Assembly of National Voluntary Health and Social Welfare Organizations, 1993

Chapter.....3

Groundwork to Stimulate Local Political Will for Change

- Why Political Will?

- Tools and Strategies to Stimulate Political Will for Changes in Local Health Care

WHY POLITICAL WILL?

For a community to successfully conceive of and implement an effective strategy for its uninsured, there must be widespread political will, both among the general population and within the numerous groups of stakeholders. By "political will" we mean a conscious resolve to effect change, which the community is willing to apply to the ways its individual and collective stakeholders allocate resources and make decisions.

Without corresponding political will, provider-driven approaches to the uninsured are rarely effective. Providers appear greedy and are not able to generate consensus and support among the other stakeholders for the strategies they propose. "Professional will" cannot replace grassroots political will. The consensus-building process used to generate political will validates the common concerns shared between members of the professional, business, and lay community sectors and educates members of the professional and business sectors about the lay community's attitudes and wishes. Generating political will is a crucial step in building the underpinnings needed for effective community problem solving.

TOOLS AND STRATEGIES TO STIMULATE POLITICAL WILL FOR CHANGE

The best tools to assess and marshal political will are opinion polls, surveys, public forums, private forums, and media coverage — all tools commonly used in the political process to gather, produce, and use information with a desired outcome in mind.

Gathering Information About Your Community

Your Steering Committee's first step toward generating political will should be to gather detailed information about your community's population and the opinions of residents and stakeholder groups. Essentially, you will need to create a snapshot of your community as it exists.

We use the terms assessment, survey, poll, and study interchangeably for these activities. Inventory, survey, or polling strategies will help you understand exactly how the various subgroups in your community feel about, and have experienced, the issues of lack of health insurance or lack of access to health care services.

Your assessment should pose a variety of questions, some lengthy, to determine community members' understanding of the issue, how important the issue is to them, and how strong their will to change the situation is. You should intentionally over-sample certain minority groups to help you gain a solid view of these individuals' perspectives and to engage them in the assessment process in meaningful ways. It is important that your assessment identifies what opinions or perspectives are held widely enough that they can be defined as community priorities and serve as community-wide rallying points to unify members of your community and inspire them to work toward your goals.

Your Steering Committee also should collect data that will enable planners and implementers to target discrete parts of the community. Subgroups can be identified by age, by neighborhood, by gender, by occupation, by income level, and by many other factors.

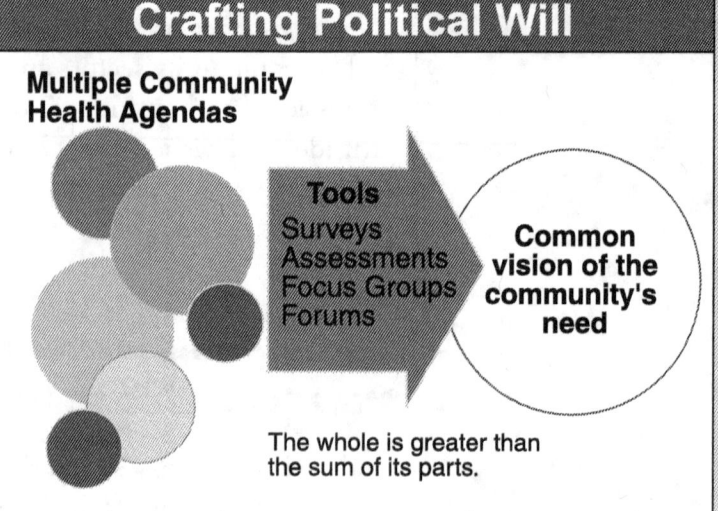

Cross-tabulations (the basic units of analysis within a survey or study) can be combined for comparative analysis and can provide you with astonishing detail about how members of your community's sub-groups feel. For example, cross-tabs would allow you to compare how women over age 40, registered Republicans within a particular zip code, and men who have been uninsured perceive lack of insurance. Designing the appropriate cross-tabs to meet your needs is extremely important. A community-wide assessment can provide information about segments of the population such as:

· Whether or not they understand who is uninsured and why;

· How they view the issue of lack of insurance from social and business perspectives;

- Whether they have been uninsured, and what that was like;

- Whether they accurately understand the problems faced by the uninsured portion of their own population segment;

- How they rank certain elements of health insurance (i.e., as very important, somewhat important, neutral, or unimportant);

- Where they go for information; and

- Who they trust in the community, and why.

In designing your study instrument(s), take the time to look at some of the recent national studies on the uninsured, such as the new national census data and surveys conducted by the Urban Institute, the Kaiser Family Foundation, and other organizations. Also look for state-based studies that have been done in your own state. When you review these studies, be on the lookout for questions you can use in your own study instruments. By repeating some of the questions from these other instruments, you will be able to assess your community's standing compared to national or state norms.

Develop, administer, and analyze your assessment quickly, then present your analysis of the results in ways that all stakeholders will find useful and easy to understand. Design simple graphs, charts, and trend lines. Avoid presenting table after table of data or using statistical jargon that people may not understand. Remember: at this point, you are providing *information*, not solutions.

Finding Technical Assistance

Well-defined and accurate baseline data will form the foundation of your community's efforts. Therefore, it is wise to seek technical assistance in designing your community's survey instruments, conducting the inventory, and analyzing and reporting the data.

Most communities have access to consultants who have expertise in all these areas; health care expertise is less important than experience with survey instruments and analyzing opinion data. Universities and colleges are one resource that can be tapped for this technical assistance; so are private consulting firms. You also may want to use the expertise of a political polling firm, particularly one that employs non-partisan strategies.

When choosing a consultant, look for someone who is neutral on your issues (i.e., that doesn't have a prearranged agenda) and credible in your community. Your consultant should be able to show you how he or she has been able to present findings in user-friendly, easy-to-understand formats for other clients. Your consultant also should clearly understand that your goal is to gather real-time, accurate data to produce a snapshot of your community – not to conduct a long-term research study.

ACTION TIPS

Objectives for This Step

1. Identify similarities and differences in the ways various sectors of your community (e.g., employed versus unemployed people and members of various racial, age, or political groups) perceive the uninsured. Try to determine why they feel that way.

2. Identify issues of consensus that can serve as rallying points to generate political will for change.

3. Identify issues and means that you can use to target your education and advocacy efforts to certain subgroups of your community and also to communicate to the entire community at once.

Organizing

During the process of creating your community-wide snapshot, your Steering Committee should continue to act as the focal point for organizing and decision-making. We recommend that you also create a subcommittee to develop your assessment instrument in conjunction with the organization you select to conduct it. Members are likely to be a mix of Steering Committee members and other people with survey expertise. This subcommittee should be in charge of coordinating the development, use, and analysis of your survey. The subcommittee also should oversee the comparison of your survey results with results of other surveys and should help compile a presentation of your completed

In Muskegon County, 97 percent of those people surveyed agreed that children should have access to health care regardless of their ability to pay. That became the "rallying point" around which we built political will we could harness for change.

findings and analysis to the full Steering Committee and other interested stakeholders.

Decision Making

Decisions should continue to be consensus-driven at this point. Members of your Steering Committee should be involved and should agree on all the "big picture" decisions for this venture (e.g., the broad elements and objectives of the initial study, how to present the findings of the initial survey, and what should happen next).

Your Steering Committee will need to make decisions about:

· Which population sub-groups need accurate education about the uninsured;

· Which subgroup leaders need to be engaged, at what point they need to be engaged, and how to engage them;

In Muskegon County, we found large differences in how the uninsured were perceived by different constituencies, such as union members and small business owners. Our poll also sought information about insurance copays as barriers to care and other access issues. We found that most of our uninsured were women who were under the age of 40, had children, and were employed in service or retail sectors. We also found that 75 percent of our African-American residents felt our community needed more minority physicians.

· The most effective ways to engage the right people in your process; and

· Who in the Steering Committee will be charged with each step.

Who Pays for This Step?

A community-wide study will cost money. Ideally, your Steering Committee will be able to pool as much as $25,000 to complete this step. But, from where?

While 'planning money' is hard to find these days, there may be local resources (e.g., county government, local corporate or community foundations) that can be tapped. Local businesses, United Ways, or health systems also may be willing to fund all or part of this effort. Because of their interest in this topic, local newspapers may be willing to underwrite some or all of this work, too, so don't be afraid to ask them.

A less expensive (but less complete) strategy is to tack your questions onto surveys or questionnaires that already are in progress in your community, such as those routinely conducted by hospitals, newspapers, local public health departments, and other organizations.

Record Keeping

As in the previous step, you will need accurate records of decisions so you can document the consensus-building process and establish credibility. Decisions will be made about who will design your instruments, who will conduct and analyze the data, where resources will come from, and timelines for completion of various steps. It is very important that you produce and circulate timely, formal, decision-based minutes and attendance records throughout the process.

Tips for Conveners

The Steering Committee convener has a challenge. He/she needs to facilitate all the necessary meetings to create a polling instrument, process the polling data, and prepare to move to the next step (i.e., selecting targeted issues for action).

Every one of these tasks produces tangible results, which make the Steering Committee feel satisfied and productive. But, at the same time, the convener must be sure to allow enough time for the Steering Committee to embrace ownership and investment in the process and its products, and not feel forced or manipulated.

The convener must artfully juggle process and outcome, trust and productivity.

Hazards and Traps

- "Analysis Paralysis" is common at this point. The temptation to collect more data — to look deeper before taking decisive action — can stall, and eventually kill groups. Your inventory will give you plenty of information upon which to act.

- Fear of baseline data also can be a problem. Some stakeholders may be reluctant to take a clear snapshot of community perceptions, because they fear what it might show. Be brave!

- Another hazard is the temptation to craft your own survey or poll, without working with someone who has proven survey expertise. The professional quality of your assessment and its analysis are crucial. Spend the money now, and save it on some other steps later.

- "Going public" too early is another hazard that should be avoided. While the data that you collect is by no means secret, the timing of its widespread release is crucial. At this stage, it is best to avoid a media blitz, which is likely to sensationalize data, rather than put it to constructive use.

- Allow members of your Steering Committee enough time to make this process their own. Don't adopt someone else's survey to save time; don't jam data or implementation plans down people's throats. Ownership and personal investment are important; support a process that builds this investment.

- Finally, remember that too much process without results will make your Steering Committee members feel they are wasting their time.

Additional Resources

Families USA
(www.familiesusa.org) 1334 G. St, N.W., Washington D.C., 20005
Phone 202-628-3030, Fax 202-347-2417

Kaiser Family Foundation
(www.kff.org) 2400 Sand Hill Rd, Menlo Park, CA 94025
Phone 650-854-9400, Fax 650-854-4800

National Governor's Association
(www.nga.org) Hall of States, 444 N. Capitol St., Washington
D.C., 20001-1512
Phone 202-624-5300

W.K. Kellogg Foundation
(www.wkkf.org) One Michigan Ave. East, Battle Creek, MI 49017
Phone 616-968-1611, Fax 616-968-0413

Commonwealth Fund
(www.cmwf.org) One East 75th St., New York, NY 10021
Phone 212-606-3800, Fax 212-606-3500

Robert Wood Johnson Foundation
(www.rwjf.org) P.O. Box 2316, College Rd, East and Route 1
Princeton, NJ 08543-2316
Phone 1-888-631-9989

Welfare Info Network
(www.welfareinfo.org) 1000 Vermont Ave., N.W., Suite 600
Washington D.C., 20005
Phone 202-628-5790, Fax 202-268-4206

The Access Project
(www.accessproject.org) 30 Winter St, Suite 930
Boston, MA 02108
Phone 617-654-9911, Fax 617-654-9922

American Academy of Family Physicians
(www.aafp.org) 11400 Tomahawk Creek Parkway
Leawood, KS 66211-2672
Phone 913-906-6000

Chapter.....4

Build and Use a Legitimate Community-Driven Engine for Change

- Decide On a Governance Model

- The Governing Body's Objectives and Strategies

- The Community-Based Work Teams' Objectives and Strategies

At this point, your original Steering Committee has good information about who is uninsured in your community, how your community views the uninsured, and how lack of health insurance and other access issues impact community residents, schools, businesses, and service organizations. You also know which health issues are the most sensitive in your community, and to whom. You have identified several key problems that are not being addressed to the community's satisfaction; some are widespread and others impact certain community segments. Now it is time to reorganize in order to act on that information.

Several key organizational factors are crucial at this point:

- The Steering Committee needs to migrate to a more formal governance structure;

- Community-based action teams need to be fostered and supported;

- All parties at all levels need to commit to true community-based, bottom-up, local solutions; and

- The governing body and the action teams need integrated processes through which they will communicate regularly so their work will be well-coordinated and will effectively serve the community.

DECIDE ON A GOVERNANCE MODEL

Until now, your Steering Committee has driven the processes of data collection, analysis, and sharing with the community. Now, it is time to migrate to a more formal, public, and accountable structure. The governance model you select is less important than assurance that it has certain critical factors. To be successful, your governance model must:

- Have credibility as a neutral body;

- Be vested with the authority to get things done;

- Have a broad and representative membership;

- Be capable of performing fiduciary functions; and

· Be "branded" with a recognizable name and mission.

Neutral means that there is no preconceived program or product on the part of the group. While there may be members who act from enlightened self-interest, the group itself will be accountable to ensure that no one member or subset of members railroads the process. The interest of the community at large must be the governing body's focus. When an organization or special interest begins to assert undue influence on your process, your group must redirect itself back to its broader common agenda.

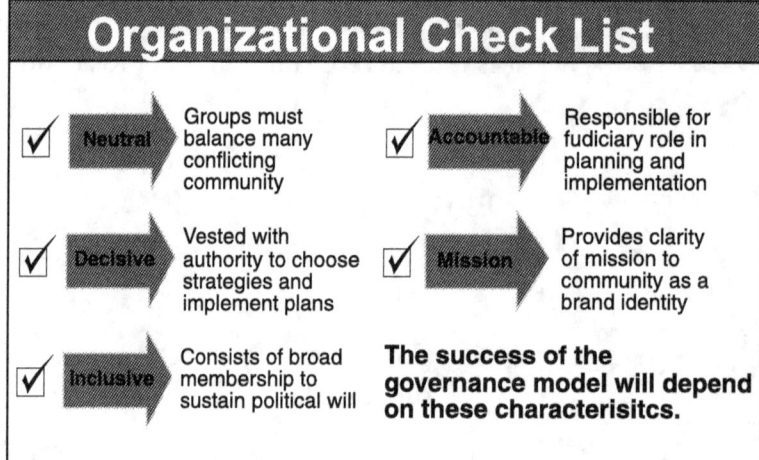

Vested with authority means the members of your governing body must be decision-makers and people with significant influence in your community. While your governing body itself will not identify specific change strategies, it will use its influence to garner resources, facilitate policy changes, influence the media, and take other steps to bring the action plans of the community action teams to life.

Broad and representative membership means there must be representation not just from the obvious health-related players, but also from key minorities, businesses, schools, faith-based organizations, and safety net organizations in your community.

The governing body's *fiduciary function* is key; its role will include collecting and distributing resources to the community action teams, as well as accounting for the use of the resources. It must have the capacity to carry out these financial functions in a timely and accountable manner.

A recognizable "brand" and mission is key to a successful effort. Your governing group, and the community action teams that function under its direction, must become a visible, recognizable

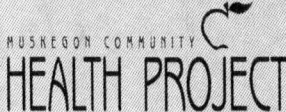
force within your community. For this to happen, you will need a "brand" (a name that is recognizable), as well as a short, concise mission statement that can be remembered easily and repeated all over town. Even if you decide that a single organization will house your governing body, you still must make certain that your effort has a broader identity. Find a brand name for yourselves, and make it a catchy one.

There are many ways your governing body can organize. Your job will be to go back to your stakeholder analysis and identify the type of structure that is most appropriate for your situation. You probably will be able to identify several organizations in your community that could serve as a parent to the governing body, and some of those organizations may have affiliate national organizations that also support community health improvement. Such organizations may include:

· Your local chamber of commerce;

· Your local public health department;

· Your local or regional health alliance;

· Your local United Way organization;

· Your county medical society;

· Your local hospital(s) or health system(s);

· Your local community foundation(s); and

· Your local Healthy Community coalition.

These organizations should already have the capacity to serve the required fiduciary function. Using any of them as the "parent" for your efforts will save time and, assuming that they are sufficiently neutral, lend credibility to your efforts.

Other options exist. For instance, you may choose to form a separate 501(c)(3) corporation. You also may want to consider a looser affiliation or partnership, a set-up that also is appropriate and quite manageable, if fiduciary obligations are clear.

In seating this governing body, you will need to address all of the issues of starting a new group — membership rules, operational ground rules, decision-making processes, meeting locations, communications, and more. There are many resources and consultants available to support you in these important steps, and you also have people in your community who are experienced and available to help. Don't skip over the steps of defining these critical rules and processes; take the time to create a solid foundation.

Be sure to build in staff support to the governing body, as well as clear lines of responsibility and funding for that support. As the governance becomes more formal, so must the clerical and professional support of the governance.

Finally, in developing your governing body's ground rules, be sure to take time to address the fundamentals of community-driven change. Make sure the members of your governing body understand and are committed to bottom-up, locally driven solutions, and that they are prepared to accept the community action teams' recommendations. *There is no role for the governing body to undo and redo the work of the community action teams.*

THE GOVERNING BODY'S OBJECTIVES AND STRATEGIES

The new Governing Body has four overarching objectives at this point:

1. To stimulate the community's political will to address its uninsured;

2. To launch multiple investigations into areas of concern;

3. To support community-based action teams in their processes to investigate issues and explore solutions; and

4. To interface with community-based action teams in ways that facilitate integration and sharing of information.

Organizing to meet these objectives will give structure to the governing body's meetings and help create and sustain momentum. Each objective has its own strategies, described below. Communication is an underlying function of the governing role, and you will notice that each strategy includes a strong communication component, either with the community at large or among and between the work groups.

Strategies to Stimulate Political Will

Your steering committee already has conducted a comprehensive community poll with numerous cross-tabs, and has identified issues of concern within the community, as well as natural "rallying points." Now, your original steering committee members need to bring the rest of the new governing body up to speed. This is the time for them to share the polling instrument and the results, and to

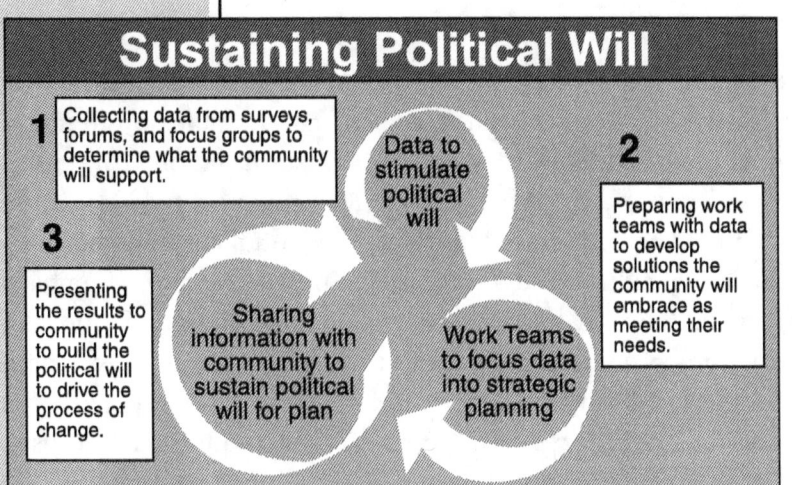

answer any questions the new governing body may have about them. Now also is the time when all those involved must agree upon which issues are the natural bases for concern and action in your community.

Armed with the data from these decisions, it is time to present what you have discovered to the public and support the formation of issue-specific action teams. Remember: you still are building awareness and political will, and political-style tools still are

For us, the issue of dental services for children showed up in our poll data and at the public hearings. Mothers shared their frustrations at finding services for their children's rotting teeth, and Head Start administrators told of their impending disqualification from state funds because they couldn't get the required dental assessments for their kids. No one had appreciated the scope of this access problem before these hearings. A head of steam quickly formed, and it was soon clear that this was an issue that should be tackled early and with vigor.

effective.

One effective strategy you can use to engage members of your community is the community forum or public hearing. A "Mayor's Forum" or other non-partisan gathering (or series of gatherings) is an excellent vehicle. You will want the media to help publicize the event, and to attend it and report on it.

In Muskegon County, our poll showed us that our African-American community was not familiar with the depth of its health problems. Our data showed much higher levels of uninsurance and lower levels of health status among this group than anyone expected. We convened ten African-American community leaders, and our public health department showed them their data. A second, larger gathering was held a few weeks later. We didn't need to convene a third — by then, members of the African-American community had become angered and energized, and they were ready to take action. From that point forward, our efforts supported theirs. Several specific health-related African-American initiatives took shape, as independent yet integrated efforts with our larger efforts to address the uninsured, and the African-American community remained heavily involved in designing our health coverage product.

Promote the fact that you will be sharing data from your community survey, as well as asking those in attendance to come forward and share their feelings and experiences related to what you have found. A credible, neutral spokesperson should present your findings, and a skilled facilitator should oversee the public comment portion of your meeting(s).

Meeting(s) such as this offer a powerful way to gather qualitative, experiential information that will validate the quantitative data your poll produced and put a face on the uninsured in your community. Remember, it is important to tend to the "human side of the equation."

Some of the issues that arise from the results of your community survey may require a more targeted approach. For instance, you may find several main issues, each of which impacts just one portion of your population, such as the elderly or a particular ethnic group. In those cases, you will want to go directly to a group of potential leaders from the affected population to present the data and build understanding and political will.

To do this, you will need to select a neutral, credible person from the governing body to convene the small group. In your first meeting, you need only to share what you have found. In a second gathering, the leaders and convener can share what initiatives are already underway to address the issue, bring supplemental qualitative or quantitative data, brainstorm, or even all three. Often, that's all it takes to fire up a group.

Strategies to Launch Multiple Investigations Into Areas of Concern

Let's assume that you now have several large and small groups that are fired up about specific issues. At this point, it is appropriate for your governing body to formally acknowledge these groups as community-based action teams, and invite them to drill down into their specific local health care access issues, and craft interventions to address them.

The strategy is not difficult — simply make certain that the action teams understand the governing structure and, where possible, ask that a member of the governing body be directly involved with each of the action teams. That ensures good exchange of information between the governing body and the action teams, as well as between the individual action teams. Also, this will enable people on the governing body to have a real-time awareness as the community efforts take shape, greatly reducing surprises and disagreements that could occur later in the process.

Your governing body's task is to publicly acknowledge all of the action teams and to lay out structures and processes to capture their recommendations. While it is *not* possible to dictate how long it will take for an action team to craft a local solution to an issue, it *is* appropriate to ask for periodic written updates and presentations at governing body meetings. This is important for cross-pollination of ideas and data, as well as in maintaining momentum. Governing body meetings must include updates on each recognized activity so its members are aware of the directions and shapes that come from the action groups and, therefore, can be supportive of the action groups' recommendations.

In addition, it is essential that your governing body appoint a

It is essential that your governing body appoint a specific group of people to further study the local uninsured issue in detail, to provide accurate data about who is currently uninsured and under-insured, why, and the projected trends for both groups.

specific group of people to further study the local uninsured issue in detail, to provide accurate data about who is currently uninsured and under-insured, why, and the projected trends for both groups. If an action team has not naturally coalesced around this issue, your governing body must assign the task to an action team. This action team must fulfill specific responsibilities, which will be detailed in the next chapter.

Strategies to Support Community-Based Action Teams

It is the role of your governing body to support the action teams. "Support" can be given in a variety of ways. For instance, organizations on the governing body can allow teams to meet in their facilities, providing meeting space and refreshments. Support with clerical functions is also key — assigning a secretary to do mailings, arrange meetings, and prepare meeting materials is very valuable to volunteer community-based action teams.

Through its members' relationships and the power of their connections in the community, your governing body also can provide community-based action teams with access to policy makers, sources of data, members of the media, and other valuable tangible and intangible resources.

The governing body's role is to use what it has to support the action teams in accomplishing their objectives. It is understood that the governing body will do this *without trying to influence the action teams' recommendations.* Again, neutrality on the part of the governors and demonstrated support of bottom-up efforts are essential.

Strategies to Facilitate Integration and Sharing of Information

The last function of the governing

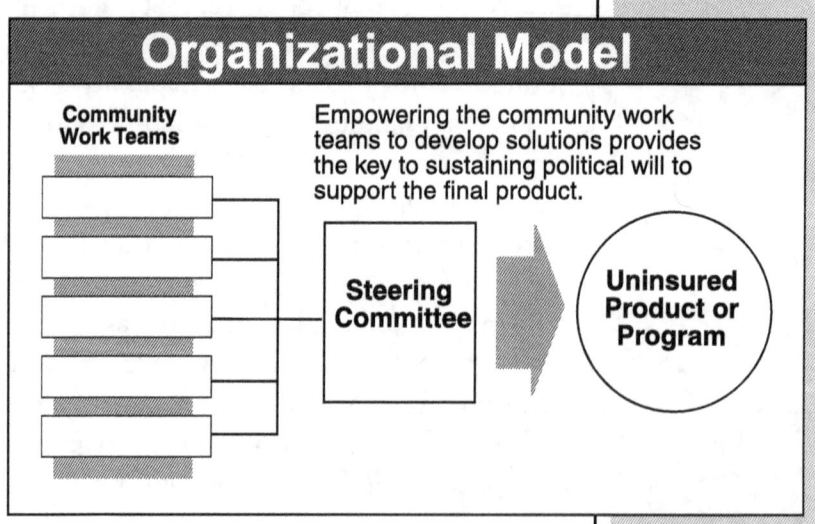

Organizational Model

Community Work Teams

Empowering the community work teams to develop solutions provides the key to sustaining political will to support the final product.

Steering Committee

Uninsured Product or Program

body at this juncture is to provide the structure through which all the parties communicate. Your governing body should meet regularly and focus on supporting your community action teams. It should stay apprised of action teams' activities and provide opportunities for the teams to hear from one another. This is a dynamic, interactive process. It cannot be rushed, and it should not be forced.

Over the course of months, members of your action teams and governing body will become more familiar with one another, and more informed about health issues in your community. At some point, a vision for your community will emerge. It is your governing body's responsibility to facilitate the emergence of this common vision, raise it up the flag pole, and then garner the resources to achieve it.

THE COMMUNITY-BASED ACTION TEAMS' OBJECTIVES AND STRATEGIES

Each community-based action team has three overarching objectives:

1. Study the issue at hand in detail;

2. Report findings and recommendations to the governing body and fellow action teams over time; and

3. Assist in implementation of the chosen activities.

Organizing to meet these objectives will give structure to the action teams and create and sustain momentum. Each objective has its own strategies, described below.

Strategies to Study the Issue in Detail

Here, each action team drills deeply and comprehensively to confirm the impact of its issue on the community (including individuals, providers, businesses, safety net groups, schools, churches, and others), and to document the existing situation. The team will study its own assets and deficits and be self-directed in developing solutions for the issues it holds dear.

The time and resources required for this step will vary widely, but the task is the same. A forced time structure will sabotage this work, but it is appropriate to identify the expected outcomes and ask for regular updates.

Strategies to Report Findings and Recommendations

Each action team needs to remain in communication with the governing body and with the other action teams. High-quality communication and cross-fertilization also occurs when a governing body member belongs to (or is assigned to) each action team.

The action teams need to process their findings and come forward with realistic, achievable recommendations. Your governing body may wish to ask for recommendations in a common form (i.e., that each team report its work using a common outline or format). Your governing body should remind action teams that their recommendations should address resource requirements, too. No team should expect that its recommendations will be funded by the governing body.

Strategies to Implement Recommendations

Keep in mind that each action team will include participants who can only be involved in the effort for the short term. (That pesky day job does have its obligations.) However, it will have others who are able to remain active for the long haul.

As your community moves into the implementation phase, it will need to reorganize once again. But, it is important that each initiative includes at least a few people who were involved in the research and design phase; those people bring history and continuity to the teams, and they represent the original intent of the effort. Effective bottom-up solutions include community-based champions in design *and* implementation.

ACTION TIPS

So, you have built a legitimate community-driven engine for change, and are using it to find your community's vision for health. Here are some issues you are guaranteed to bump into.

Decision Making

Regardless of your best efforts, someone is guaranteed to try to scuttle the bottom-up model by manipulating the decision-making process. Don't be surprised when it happens, but don't let the culprit get away with it, either.

The culprit may be a hospital CEO, a hospital board member, or a hospital staff person who gets nervous when it looks like an action team may want the hospital to deliver free services. It may be one or more members of an action team who are especially adept at advocacy and want to hog the resources. Be on guard, and remind your governing body that it is everyone's duty to speak against bullying.

Who Pays for This Step?

As mentioned earlier, there may be planning money available from a variety of sponsors for this work. Then again, there may not be.

Part of your governing body's role is to scare up resources through its members' connections. Action teams, too, will have unique ideas and resources for funding their individual efforts. The key is to coordinate it all so that every action team can meet its objectives, if possible. It's a challenge.

Record Keeping

Your governing body must maintain accurate records. Formal decision-based minutes and attendance records must be produced and circulated.

The harder task may be convincing the community action teams that they must maintain accurate records, too. Remind them that in every step, precise records of decisions are crucial in documenting the consensus-building process and in establishing credibility.

Again, your governing body may wish to provide clerical support to the action teams to help them in this function; your help will almost always be welcome.

Hazards and Traps

- Process is key. It is also slow, and some people (and groups) will buck it. Stay focused on the process, and require that all the action teams participate in it. Resist the urge to jump to solutions. You may need to call upon special facilitating skills to keep task-oriented members engaged; there are resources and consultants with the expertise to guide you through this touchy situation, if necessary.

- There will be temptation to force solutions on the community-based action teams, or to twist the teams' recommendations. Resist them! Allow the community-based teams to find their own way and make their own recommendations. Even if their recommendations are the same ones you would have made six months earlier, the important thing is that the community owns them now. That means they will have the full force of the community's support, which has everything to do with effective implementation and sustainability. Be patient, and believe in the process.

Resources

Consultants may be especially useful in setting up and launching your governing body. During this process might be a wise time to use an outside resource, who could jump-start your group and provide bylaws, operating rules, and other pieces of infrastructure much more quickly than if you did it yourselves.

Additional Resources

"Partners in Community Health" Milbank Memorial Foundation,
(www.milbank.org)
645 Madison Avenue, 15th Floor
New York, NY 10022-1095
Phone 212-355-8400 Fax 212-355-8599

"Principles of Community Engagement" Public Health
Policy & Practice Office, Centers for Disease Control and
Prevention, *(www.cdc.gov.phppo.pce)*
1600 Clifton Road
Atlanta, GA 30333
Phone 404-639-3311

National Association of County and City Health Officers,
(www.naccho.org)
1100 17th Street, Second Floor
Washington DC 20036
Phone 202-783-5550 Fax 202-783-1583

Healthcare Forum, *(www.healthonline.com)*
5575 Sterrett Place, Suite 250
Columbia, MD 21044-2682
Phone 800-463-6482 Fax 410-772-5083

Coalition for Healthier Cities and Communities,
(www.healthycommunities.org)
One N. Franklin Ave.
Chicago, IL 60606
Phone 312-422-2624 Fax 312-442-4568

"Community Initiatives for the Uninsured: How Far Can
Innovative Partnerships Take Us?" New York Academy of
Medicine, August 2000.
(www.nyam.org)
Division of Health and Science Policy,
Office of Urban Populations
1216 Fifth Avenue
New York, NY 10029
Phone 212-882-7303, Fax 212-822-7369

Chapter.....5

Understanding Your Community's Uninsured and Under-Insured

- Overview of Insured and Uninsured Populations
- The Insurance Continuum

Chapter Four noted that your community-driven change "machinery" must include an action group charged with collecting and presenting comprehensive information about the people who are uninsured and under-insured in your community. This chapter will provide a general overview of the uninsured and under-insured and will outline the objectives and steps that must be taken by the action team collecting and presenting information about these groups.

First, expect some resistance from members of your governing body to a comprehensive study of the uninsured. The providers, especially hospitals and safety net services, may object to "yet another look," claiming they already know all there is to know about the uninsured. However, the scope of this information gathering is much wider than how much uncompensated care is delivered, and a comprehensive study is essential.

Another common tendency is to lump all people with little or no insurance into one group. In fact, many subgroups exist, and each group has different economic situations, behaviors, and perspectives on health care. After studying your population in detail, you will be able to differentiate and understand the needs of people in the subgroups of your community's uninsured and under-insured.

In Muskegon, we found that per-member, per-month pharmacy costs were $8.50 for the working uninsured, and $64.00 for the indigent uninsured. This illustrates the degree to which the groups differ. Wraparound, comprehensive safety net services are essential in the high-cost indigent uninsured population, while the problems faced by the working uninsured call for altogether different strategies.

As discussed in Chapter One, the issue of health insurance (or lack of it) has social, economic, and business implications that are closely intertwined. The charge of the action group collecting and presenting comprehensive information about the uninsured and under-insured in your community is to carefully examine the different insured and uninsured sectors of your community, predict trends in movements from one sector to another, and describe the anticipated implications to the business, provider, and social stakeholders.

Where will you get this information? A good place to start is your community's 2000 census data — look for shifts and trends in population groups. Other data will be available through surveys and tracking systems already in place through local Chambers of Commerce, insurers, or advocacy groups. The rest you will need to collect along with your other assessments.

OVERVIEW OF INSURED AND UNINSURED POPULATIONS

Think of your community as comprised of a continuum of groups of people with varying degrees of health insurance coverage. Each "sector" of the continuum receives health care in some form, and some organization or individual pays for that health care. People in your community move from one sector to another, depending upon their employment, their entitlement eligibility, the availability of private insurance, and other issues.

How Change in One Sector Can Affect Another

In Muskegon County, we noted multi-year, double-digit increases in health insurance premiums for small employers, a situation that resulted in small employers shifting premiums to employees (many of whom could not afford them) or dropping health insurance coverage.

Many of these employees and their families began using safety net services for the first time, creating unanticipated waiting lists and burdens of care on the safety net providers. Many also delayed their health care or simply did not seek treatment, especially for behavioral health services. Emergency room use increased, causing hardship for the individuals, who could not pay the ER bills, and the hospitals, whose uncompensated care levels rose without warning.

Also, while there were Medicaid benefits available to many of these employees, the businesses did not have that information to share with them. We discovered a group of Medicaid-eligible residents who were not connected to any outreach network and had little chance of discovering their eligibility.

Predicting insurance trends and understanding their implications for providers and payers is the most important element in your ability to design a viable local strategy for the uninsured individuals in your community.

It is important to recognize that each time there is a significant shift from one sector to another, not only are the individuals affected, but so are the providers and the payers in the sector to which the individuals have moved.

This is a key planning issue. Careful scrutiny of the demographic and economic trends in your community will help you predict the insurance trends and understand the implications of those trends for the provider and payer groups. Predicting insurance trends and understanding their implications for providers and payers is the most important element in your ability to design a viable local strategy for the uninsured individuals in your community.

THE INSURANCE CONTINUUM

Group #1: Individuals with Commercial Insurance

- These individuals receive health insurance through employer-based plans, in which the employers pay the health insurance premiums for their employees and/or retirees.

The Continuum of Care

Medicaid	Medicare	Commercial Coverage	Working Uninsured	Indigent Coverage
Need for access to care	Need for long-term care & drug cost relief	Need lower premiums Need better coverage for the under-insured	Need for affordable coverage Resists any welfare type solution	Need case management

Changes to any part of the continuum will impact the resources available to the other parts.

- Typically, the providers for individuals in this group are the local or regional private primary and specialty care systems that contract with third-party payers.

- The payers are employers and the individuals themselves. Insured individuals pay a portion of the insurance premiums and also the portion of copays and deductibles required by the employer.

- Coverage levels vary with employer and insurance plan and are changing rapidly across the country. The current tight labor market provides an incentive for employers to continue to cover health care insurance as an employee recruitment and retention tool. However, the rising costs of plan administration, insurance premiums, and pharmaceuticals are creating pressures to either raise employees' copays or reduce coverage.

Individuals with Commercial Insurance: Trends to Identify

- How many employers are adding or removing health insurance as an employee benefit?

- Which employers, in terms of business size and wage ranges, are adding and which are removing health insurance?

- What are the trends in benefit design? (e.g., What is covered? How are premiums, copays, and deductibles handled?) Are there trends among certain types or sizes of employers? In particular, what are the behavioral health and pharmacy benefit trends?

- Where is the projected business growth in your community? Projected business reduction? What will be the impact of these trends on health insurance coverage?

> Trends to watch closely include:
> - Changes in behavioral health benefits;
> - Changes in pharmacy benefits; and
> - Shifts from defined benefits to defined contributions.

- What, if any, provider *reimbursement* issues are attached to employer-sponsored health insurance issues? How will the trends you are projecting impact the providers?

- What, if any, provider *access* issues are attached to employer-sponsored health insurance issues? How will the trends you are projecting impact the providers?

Group #2: The Under-Insured

- These people have health insurance in some form. However, the level of coverage is so limited and/or the out-of-pocket expenses are so high that these individuals cannot afford to seek timely health care prevention, diagnosis, or treatment services.

Debts pile up quickly when an illness or accident occurs to people with limited or no health care insurance. Rates of personal bankruptcy are rising as employer-based health insurance diminishes, and you should watch for this trend in your community. Personal bankruptcy creates financial and quality-of-life stressors that are manifested within communities in many ways.

- The providers of choice for individuals in this group are family doctors of many years or providers assigned by their insurance. However, economics push this population to local free or sliding-scale safety net providers, a situation that places unanticipated (and unfunded) demands on these providers.

- The payers for this group are employers and the individuals themselves. Individuals often pay a significant portion of insurance premiums, as well as copays and deductibles, as required by their plans.

- Coverage levels vary with employer and insurance plans, and may include only catastrophic care. Increasing copays (especially for pharmacy benefits) and high deductibles are characteristic, as are the absences of dental or vision benefits and severe limitations on behavioral health benefits.

The Under-Insured: Trends to Identify

- What demographics apply to those individuals you identify as being under-insured?

- Where do the under-insured seek care, what type of care do they seek, and what type of care do they delay?

- How do the under-insured pay for their care? What are the impacts on the individuals and the providers?

- What are the trends in benefit design? (e.g., What is covered? How are premiums, copays, and deductibles handled?) Are there trends among certain types or sizes of employers? In particular, what are the behavioral health and pharmacy benefit trends?

Group #3: The Working Uninsured

- These people have jobs that do not include health insurance as a benefit. Most often, they are service or retail sector jobs, which also have low compensation. These individuals may also work part-time, hold more than one part-time job, and/or work odd hours.

- These people often are referred to as "the working poor." However, they do not identify themselves as "poor," which has negative connotations. These people view themselves as self-sufficient working citizens and very often do not want government services.

- The providers for this group may be local emergency rooms, private physicians, urgent care centers, local public health departments, or other sliding-fee providers.

- The payers for this sector include providers that deliver uncompensated care, funders of local subsidized services through a safety net system, and the individuals themselves.

- This population tends to delay treatment based upon their economic constraints.

- This population may qualify for government-sponsored benefits, but may be unwilling to use them.

The Working Uninsured: Trends to Identify

- Numbers of working uninsured and their demographics (e.g., age, employment, education, and income).

- Average length of time these individuals have been without insurance.

- Patterns of health care within this group. (e.g., Where do they go for care? What health issues are they able to address, and what issues are they not able to address?)

- Eligibility for entitlement services and trends in their use.

- Provider issues with compensation and access related to this group. (Be sure to look at behavioral health and prevention services separate from primary and urgent/emergent care needs.)

- Local employer-sponsored health insurance trends for this group.

> Many small employers can only offer insurance plans whose premiums are individually or experience rated. One case of cancer, one difficult birth, or one serious bout of depression in the ranks can drive next year's premiums completely out of reach, which means the small business is left with the choice to offer no insurance or to shut down. Faced with a situation in which employers offer no insurance but have a job available, employees almost always choose a job without insurance over no job and no insurance.

Group #4: Individuals with Government-Funded, Low-Income Coverage (e.g., Medicaid, Children's Health Insurance Programs, Welfare-to-Work Programs and others)

- Each state has different eligibility and benefit structures, and it is important to completely understand your state's programs.

- The population of this group fluctuates based upon eligibility criteria; individuals may move in and out of eligibility on a monthly basis.

- The providers for this population vary widely in their receptivity and satisfaction as service providers for Medicaid beneficiaries. State-based reimbursement rates, politics, policy matters, and preferential reimbursement categories all impact a given provider group.

- "Providers" include:

  - Hospital emergency rooms, clinics, urgent care sites, and inpatient facilities;

  - Dentists;

  - Private physicians (both individuals and groups);

- Local public health departments;

- Federally Qualified Health Centers, Rural Health Clinics, and Indian Health Services;

- Safety net providers, such as school health clinics, community-based health centers, community mental health agencies, homeless health care programs;

- Substance abuse treatment providers; and

- Managed care organizations.

- Payers are the state and federal Medicaid programs and any provider or organization that covers either uncompensated care or a portion of costs considered underfunded by the reimbursement rates.

Individuals with Government-Funded, Low-Income Coverage: Trends to Identify

- What are the demographics of this group?

- What are the projected demographic trends for this group?

- What, if any, provider *reimbursement* issues are attached to this group? How will the trends you are projecting impact the providers?

- What, if any, provider *access* issues are attached to this group? How will the trends you are projecting impact the providers?

- What are the federal and state policy and reimbursement trends that might impact this group or the providers who serve them?

Group #5: Seniors and Other Individuals with Government-Funded Medicare Coverage

- Medicare is a federal health insurance program for people 65 years or older, certain people with disabilities, and people with permanent kidney failure treated with dialysis or a transplant. Medicare coverage is uniform across the country. Medicare has two parts — Part A, which is hospital insurance, and Part B, which is medical insurance.

- Medicare is not "means tested" — those who are eligible to receive it are entitled regardless of their income.

- Medicare does *not* cover all health care costs. It requires significant copays for inpatient admissions and premium payments for Part B coverage, and it does not generally include prescription benefits.

- Medicare does *not* cover long-term care (with the exception of short-term skilled nursing care). Many nursing home residents are both Medicare and Medicaid-eligible or become "dual eligible" as they exhaust their personal resources paying for nursing home care.

- Seniors with employer-based supplemental insurance or personal "Medigap" policies may have little or no out-of-pocket expense; other seniors may have high expenses for drugs, services, and premiums.

- Medicare beneficiaries choose their own provider, unless they belong to a Medicare HMO or have limited provider choice based upon a supplemental or Medigap policy.

- The payers are the federal government for the bulk of services, and either the individuals or supplemental insurance policies for premiums, drugs, and copays.

- Historically, Medicare payments to providers have been profitable; more recently the margins between health care costs and Medicare reimbursement (set by region and non-negotiable) have lessened. The recent Balanced Budget Amendment dramatically reduced reimbursement levels to hospitals and physicians, creating serious financial strain on providers with a heavy Medicare volume.

Individuals with Medicare Coverage: Trends to Identify

- What are the demographics of this group?

- What are the projected demographic trends for this group?

- What, if any, provider *reimbursement* issues are attached to this group? How will the trends you are projecting impact the providers?

- What, if any, provider *access* issues are attached to this group? How will the trends you are projecting impact the providers?

- What are the federal policy and reimbursement trends that might impact this group or the providers who serve them?

- How is this group managing the rising cost of pharmaceuticals?

Group #6: The Uninsured Indigent

- These people are usually unemployed. Often, they also are transient, disabled, mentally ill, and/or substance abusers.

- Your community's safety net providers support this population.

- The providers for this group often are the local emergency rooms, indigent care clinics, and other safety net providers.

- Providers include:

  - Hospital emergency rooms, clinics, urgent care sites, and inpatient facilities;

  - Local public health departments;

  - Federally Qualified Health Centers, Rural Health Clinics, and Indian Health Services;

  - Safety net providers, such as school health clinics, street clinics, and community mental health agencies; and

  - Substance abuse treatment providers.

- The payers for this group often are local health systems through uncompensated care and state or local programs and grants that fund indigent safety net services.

Safety net providers are programs that can offer services at a sliding fee to people with very low income. Safety net providers differ in each community, as do the resources with which they have to work.

Community Mental Health and Local Public Health are primarily government-funded safety net programs. United Way provides safety net services through charitable employee payroll deductions. Lions Clubs and other service organizations offer safety net services funded by dues and contributions, and many not-for-profit social service organizations offer safety net services through charitable contributions, fees, grants, and government funding.

The Uninsured Indigent: Trends to Identify

- What are the current demographics of this group?

- What are the projected demographic trends for this group?

- What, if any, provider *reimbursement* issues are attached to this group? How will the trends you are projecting impact the providers?

- What, if any, provider *access* issues are attached to this group? How will the trends you are projecting impact the providers?

- What are the federal and state policy and reimbursement trends that might impact this group or the providers who serve them?

A Final Word

Compiling this trend data will be an education for everyone involved. Your research will clearly highlight the ways that shifts in your community's population can be expected to impact the numerous health, social, and business stakeholders involved. It also will highlight where your community is the most vulnerable, and provide an excellent road map to targeted, effective community-based interventions to strengthen your local health system and provide coverage to your uninsured and under-insured.

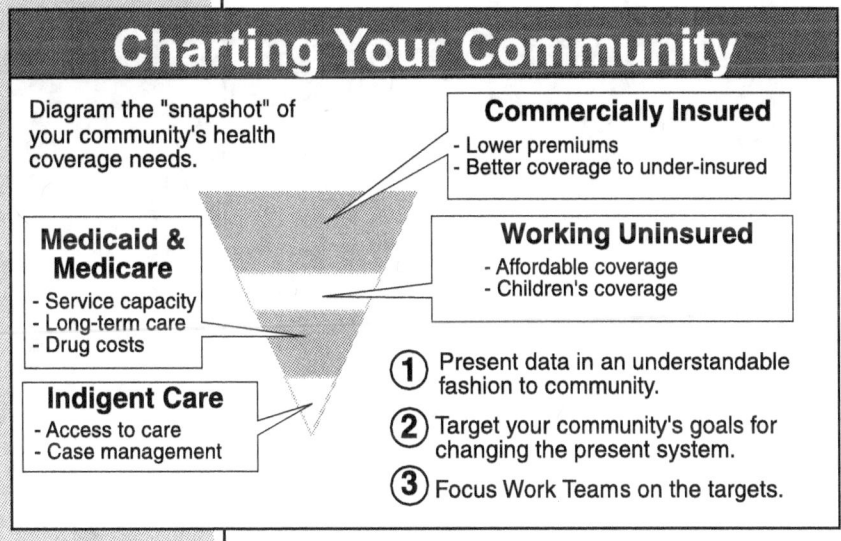

Charting Your Community

Diagram the "snapshot" of your community's health coverage needs.

Commercially Insured
- Lower premiums
- Better coverage to under-insured

Medicaid & Medicare
- Service capacity
- Long-term care
- Drug costs

Working Uninsured
- Affordable coverage
- Children's coverage

Indigent Care
- Access to care
- Case management

(1) Present data in an understandable fashion to community.

(2) Target your community's goals for changing the present system.

(3) Focus Work Teams on the targets.

Chapter.....6

Planning for Change

- Step One: Studying Successful Models

- Step Two: Selecting the Model for Your Community

- Step Three: Formalizing the Detailed Design of Your Model

This chapter will present three steps necessary to design an intervention that is right for your community. Each step is complex and requires commitment and participation from all your stakeholders. The steps are:

1. Studying the successful models from other communities to identify which approaches might be most appropriate for your situation.

2. Selecting the model you will use.

3. Formalizing the detailed design of the model, and making it your own.

STEP ONE: STUDYING SUCCESSFUL MODELS

Many communities have gone before you in creating programs and policies for their uninsured and under-insured, and there are excellent resources that will help your community quickly become familiar with the types of approaches that have worked. It is now the point in the process when you should begin an in-depth study of the array of models that can be used to address the needs of the uninsured, and to build a case for the method that will best suit your community's needs.

Your governing body will need to formally assign these tasks. Ideally, a broad-based, knowledgeable, and politically savvy ad hoc work group from your community should take on this assignment. Another option is to contract with a consultant to complete this work. (Some advice on this will follow later in the chapter.) It should be noted that this guide cannot provide all the detail you will want about particular models, but it can provide a framework with which to assess key elements that are present in each model.

Where to begin? There are many descriptions of community models available on the Internet and in books, journals, and other resources. We list plenty to get you started later in this chapter.

Framework

There are a wide variety of local programs developed for the uninsured. But any local program for the uninsured will include similar elements, and we suggest you study programs in a way that compares the variety of approaches in each element. The principal elements are:

1. Care versus coverage;

2. Continuum of services;

3. Provider payment;

4. Sources of funding; and

5. Organizational infrastructure.

Your work group or consultant should consider how the models they examine address each of these principal elements. This will create an emerging awareness of your community's situation as it relates to each of the five principal elements. In turn, it will help you identify the most feasible options for the uninsured people of your community, which ultimately will enable your community to develop its own unique model.

Element 1: Care Versus Coverage

One obvious element of a model for the uninsured is whether the program directly provides *health care services* or instead provides *financial coverage* for obtaining health care services.

Providing health care services involves designing a system of personnel and equipment to deliver that care under applicable regulations; it also might involve providing a setting in which people receive care. An example of this health care services model would be establishing an after-hours primary care clinic to detour uninsured residents from the expensive use of a local emergency room. Providing dental services using rotating volunteer dentists in a rural primary care clinic is another example.

A model that provides financial coverage for health care services does not address the delivery of health care services directly. Rather, it designs financial resources the uninsured can use to obtain health care services that already exist. An example of this approach is a model that creates a pool of funds that can be used to reimburse an existing after-hours clinic for services delivered to people whose insurance does not cover the cost of those services. Another example is the *Access Health©* model, which provides medical care coverage to uninsured employees through a shared premium structure.

There is an important distinction between *coverage* and *insurance.* Insurance products are regulated by individual states, and regulations vary widely. In general, "insurance" involves collecting premiums in exchange for a defined set of benefits, with guarantees to provide those benefits. Under insurance law, federal and state requirements related to mandatory minimum benefits and financial reserves must be met.

Usually, medical care coverage that provides dollars for services without charging premiums is not subject to such requirements, although there may be other rules that apply in your state. In some states, it is possible to charge premiums for medical care coverage without qualifying as "insurance." In Michigan, for instance, the law allows municipalities to provide such coverage. In other states, there are provisions under which the unlicensed subsidiaries of licensed insurers can provide more flexible coverage.

There is an important distinction between *coverage* and *insurance.* Insurance products are regulated by individual states, and regulations vary widely. Under insurance law, federal and state requirements related to mandatory minimum benefits and financial reserves must be met. The issues of insurance and coverage are highly complex, and you will need well-informed legal counsel to navigate this important issue.

As you study models, pay close attention to exactly what type of coverage is provided. Some models may not be applicable to your state or location, because of your state's regulation or law.

The model you select will address your community's unique service needs. You can get some ideas from the programs other communities have implemented to address the needs of their uninsured and under-insured residents.

- *Access Health* ©, in Muskegon, MI, is a fee-for-service model that provides subsidized coverage to uninsured working families for local primary, preventive and acute care.

- *Project Access* in Buncombe County, NC, connects the existing public and private health care systems with a combination of private practicing physician volunteers and donated outpatient and diagnostic services to provide the uninsured with comprehensive primary and specialty medical care.

- The *Michele Project* in Bridgeport, CT, provides mammography screening to medically underserved women, most of whom belong to a racial or ethnic minority population.

- The Minneapolis, MN, *Apple Tree Dental* project was designed to provide dental services to adults in long-term care. It has been adapted to provide dental care to other underserved populations of all ages.

- The *Bridge* program in metropolitan New York responds to significant barriers to mental health in the metropolitan Asian population by integrating mental health services with primary care for this population.

- *Project Vida* in El Paso, TX, focuses on a combination of primary health care, housing, and gang prevention for the city's indigent residents.

- The *Ingham Health Plan*, in Ingham County, MI, provides ambulatory care, including primary and specialty physician services and prescription drug coverage, to individuals with incomes less than 250 percent of poverty.

- *HealthChoice*, in Wayne County (Detroit), MI, is a managed care program that provides subsidized comprehensive health care coverage to employees, dependents, and owners of Wayne County businesses that meet program criteria.

Insufficient mental health and substance abuse services and coverage for them are extremely common problems for the uninsured and under-insured everywhere in the country.

Element 2: Continuum of Services

A model for the uninsured must determine which health care services it will address, from prevention and primary care to catastrophic care, and within the scope of physical, mental health, substance abuse, and dental services. You should now know your community's most problematic gaps in service, based upon the surveys and analyses you undertook earlier.

Programs that address financial coverage for the uninsured, like Muskegon County's *Access Health©*, also need to identify the scope of covered benefits for the areas of services being addressed.

Element 3: Provider Payment

Whether you elect a service or coverage model for your community, you will need to address both how and how much providers will be paid for the services they deliver.

Project Vida in El Paso, TX, identified one of their six key areas of concentration as "Spirit, to ensure that providers were focusing on goals, not on old feuds or avoiding risks."

The issue of provider payment is often a sensitive one, with a long history. In some communities, the sensitivity of this issue will require special handling. Familiarity with a variety of payment models will help you navigate your local discussions. Communities around the country have developed a wide diversity of provider payment models. They include:

- Donated physician, dentist, and hospital services;
- Medicaid fee screens;
- Discounted fee-for-service;
- Full capitation; and
- Cost-based reimbursement.

A variety of payment options exist and, as always, what is the most appropriate for your community depends upon your unique situation. You may also find that you can use several different approaches for different types of services.

Element 4: Sources of Funding

Communities must be very creative in deciding the source(s) from which to fund an initiative for the uninsured. Examples of what has been done include everything from new, tax-generated dollars to re-allocation of existing federal funds from the Medicaid program.

Within the element of funding, there are variables that can combine in many ways. Each variable has significance to your situation. No one source or combination of funding is inherently better than another; it is just different. Successful community interventions require a thorough understanding of the rules and implications associated with all the dollars you want to use to finance your program. The variables include:

- Local versus "external" funding;
- Private sector, nonprofit/philanthropic, or government funding;
- New versus existing funding; and
- Blended funds.

Local versus "external" funding: both local and external funds can come from private sector, not-for-profit, or government sources. The use of local funds usually implies a greater commitment to local control and innovation, long-term program success, and fewer "strings" or regulations tied to the funds. Local funding might be drawn from local employers or employee contributions, taxes, community foundations, or United Way support.

Be aware that local funds often are difficult to secure for planning and start-up activities, because community investors typically want to put their resources into programs that are up and operating. An exception may be local dollars that become available through a public or nonprofit hospital conversion, which has created a local foundation with a health care focus.

Many communities have sought money from foundations or government agencies to support their planning efforts. Foundation and governmental grants often come with programmatic strings attached, which may limit your flexibility in program design. This is particularly true in certain demonstration projects or governmental grant programs.

Private sector, nonprofit/philanthropic, or government funding: Private sector funds can come from a wide variety of sources and can be quite innovative. Examples include: premium payments from individuals; program contributions from participating businesses; direct corporate contributions; and matching funds from large employers and corporations. Private funds are usually from local or statewide sources.

Nonprofit funds/philanthropic funds can also be local, state-based, or from national or international sources. Sources would include local United Ways or other nonprofits, local, state or national foundations, or international corporate foundations.

Government funding can come from county, city, state, or federal sources. Local government support is often limited to crisis situations, but can be very handy and generous during a crisis. State and federal sources are usually tied to a policy initiative, so it is important to be connected to state and federal policy trends in order to be aware of funding opportunities.

New versus existing funding: There are many examples of communities creating new sources of revenue for their uninsured resident programs, and an equal number of programs that redirect existing revenue. New sources include taxes, fees, premium payments, and volunteer in-kind support. Existing revenue involves diverting dollars from one use to another, or combining them in new ways.

Blended funds: Many communities finance their programs by blending several sources of funding into a unique financing approach. Old, new, local, state, private, and public sector revenues can be combined creatively to produce the resources necessary to fund the desired array of services. A consideration, especially if dealing with Medicaid, is how the combination of new or existing revenue can increase the level of federal dollars that might be available to your initiative.

The "Sustainability Factor"

A word of caution: Be careful to examine the expected duration of your selected funding streams. In particular, grants, demonstration projects, or other philanthropic sources are often time-limited. Government revenues also change over time.

While no plan will have permanent funding, be careful to select financing that will sustain your initiative for the period required to make it viable on its own.

In studying the funding models of other communities, pay attention to these questions, and be prepared to identify how they apply to each source of funding:

- Who is contributing money?
- Why?
- For how long?
- What does the funder want to see as an outcome?
- When must that outcome be achieved?
- How invested is the funder in supporting local control?
- What "strings" are attached to the funds?
- What regulations apply to the funds?

Element 5: Organizational Infrastructure

No matter what your design, your initiative will need an infrastructure (permanent governance and ownership) and an accountable mechanism for reporting financial transactions, establishing contracts, collecting data, and more. The models you study will exhibit an array of infrastructure options, including 501(c)(3) organizations, units within existing organizations, public/private partnerships with a fiduciary, and many others.

In reviewing community models, your work group or consultant should pay attention to these infrastructure issues:

- The governance structure of the model, including its decision-making process and authority;

- Channels and methods of accountability to funders, stakeholders, and the public;

- The mechanisms for contracting, purchasing, marketing, hiring and managing personnel, and financing (i.e., how the daily work gets done);

- Collection and reporting of financial and utilization data; and

- Feedback mechanisms for client, provider, and funder satisfaction.

These are complex issues that will require a great deal of time and attention. The success and sustainability of your intervention is heavily dependent upon a solid, functional infrastructure that is politically and financially viable in your community. Be prepared to spend a lot of time considering your options for an infrastructure.

ACTION TIPS

Step One Objectives

Study the various successful models that other communities have used to address their uninsured and under-insured, using an organized framework. Analyze the models along their common principal elements of:

- Health care service versus payment for coverage;
- Health care service continuum;
- Provider payment;
- Funding;
- Infrastructure.

Organizing

Your governing body should appoint an ad hoc work group to conduct this analysis and assign a timeline for completion. Members should include stakeholders who not only represent a broad spectrum of the community, but who also are knowledgeable and conversant enough in health care to understand the models and contribute to the analysis.

A university, public health department, hospital, or large employer may have staff or interns they will "lend" to contribute to the data collection. A consultant also can be employed. However, be extremely cautious in selecting a consultant to ensure that you are not hiring someone who has a "canned" answer for your community. The consultant should not have his/her own product or model to sell, but should support your objective data collection and analytic processes.

Who Pays for This Step?

You may or may not need external resources for this step. If you use local individuals, their time may be contributed in-kind. If external consultants are required, you can seek funding support from individual organizations or foundations.

Another option at this point is to seek a formal grant from a local or external funder for this entire three-step portion of your process. Your governing body and work groups have built enough experience and outcomes by this point to be able to present a credible proposal. (If you decide to seek a formal grant, make sure to account for resources you will need during the detailed design phase described in Step Three.)

A note: Most of the information you need for this step is available over the Internet or through conversations with key parties around the country. You are not ready to make site visits. You may, though, wish to expose your work group to conferences or other resources on this topic.

Decision Making

There are no formal decisions to make in this step. Your governing body should provide guidance as to how many models and what types of models the work group should analyze, and the work group should create its own operating rules.

Record Keeping

The work group needs to present a clear, easy-to-understand summary of its analyses. It will need to keep records and produce presentation materials accordingly.

Hazards

- As noted previously, external consultants may come with a pre-fabricated solution to your community's situation; many firms have preferred models to sell and may not be as neutral as you would like. Select consultants carefully.

- Certain stakeholders may become anxious during this step and the ones that follow, as they may fear certain models that compete with, or compromise, their interests. You may see political maneuvering, stonewalling, and other subtle or overt signs of growing conflict. Your governing body needs to keep careful tabs on signs of conflict of interest, and manage them discreetly and effectively.

Resources

There are many sources of information on community-based initiatives to address the uninsured and under-insured. The following is not a comprehensive list, but these Internet sites are the most comprehensive and will provide you with a wealth of information and links to many other sources. You will find conference reports, descriptions of local programs, and links to program web sites, journal articles, data, contact information, and more.

U.S. Department of Health Resources and Services Administration (HRSA), HRSA, Bureau of Primary Health Care *(www.hrsa.gov)*

The Bureau's programs offer valuable information on local models. Bureau sites worth visiting include:

- The Center for Community Development
  (www.bphc.hrsa.gov/CCD/CCD1.htm)
  4350 East-West Highway, 8th Floor, Bethesda, MD 20814
  Phone 301-594-4296

- The Models That Work Campaign
  (www.bphc.hrsa.gov/mtw/)
  4350 East-West Highway, Bethesda, MD 20814
  Phone 800-859-2386

- Community Access Program *(www.hrsa.gov/CAP)*
  Parklawn Building, 5600 Fischers Lane,
  Rockville, MD 20857

- Center for Communities in Action
  (*www.bphc.hrsa.gov/campaign/)*
  4350 East-West Highway, Bethesda, MD 20814
  Phone 301-594-3802 Fax 301-594-4987

Volunteers in Health Care
  (www.volunteersinhealthcare.org) 111 Brewster St.
  Pawtucket, RI 02680 Phone 877-844-8442

This organization provides technical assistance by linking physician leaders with the tools and expertise to expand volunteer health care programs for the uninsured.

The Healthcare Forum *(www.healthonline.com)*
5575 Sterrett Place, Suite 250
Columbia, MD 21044-2682
Phone 800-463-6482, Fax 410-772-5083

The Forum is dedicated to improving health and quality of
life by developing individual, organizational and
community leadership capacities. It sponsors the
International Healthier Communities Award Program,
which showcases ideas for improving health.

The Coalition for Healthier Cities and Communities
(www.healthycommunities.org)
One N. Franklin Avenue, Chicago, IL 60606
Phone 312-422-2624, Fax 312-422-4568

The Coalition provides access to a rich learning base of
case studies, success stories, best practice information, and
more.

Apple Tree Dental *(www.appletreedental.org)* 8960
Springbrook Drive, Suite 150 Minneapolis, MN 55433, Phone
763-784-7993 Fax 763-784-5978

Project Vida *(www.pcusa.org)* Presbyterian Church USA,
100 Witherspoon Street, Louisville, KY 40202
Phone 888-728-7228, Fax 502-569-5018

Muskegon Community Health Project *(www.mchp.org)*
565 W. Western Avenue, Muskegon, MI 49440
Phone 231-728-3201

Hillsborough County *(www.hillsboroughcounty.org)* 601 E.
Kennedy Blvd., 25th Floor, Tampa, FL 33601
Phone 813-272-5040 Fax 813-272-2865

Ingham Health Plan *(www.ingham.org/hd/IHPhomepage.htm)*
PO Box 30161, Lansing, MI 48909
Phone 517-887-4311, Fax 517-887-4310

HealthChoice *(www.waynecounty.com/hcs)* 640 Temple, 3rd
Floor, Detroit, MI 48201
Phone 313-833-3450 or 1-800-WELLNOW, Fax 313-833-3429

STEP TWO: SELECTING THE MODEL FOR YOUR COMMUNITY

It's decision time! Your community needs to digest the analysis of models used by other communities, consider your unique circumstances, and identify your course of action. This will require a series of carefully organized, facilitated sessions with your Steering Committee, work and action groups, stakeholders, and the community at large.

In order to reach a community-wide decision on a tailored intervention, you will need to follow an organized process. We believe it must include each of the following components in some fashion. The formality with which each component occurs depends upon your unique community, but each is essential.

- The ad hoc work group presents its analysis of community models to the governing body, and through a guided process, the group reaches consensus on how the findings apply to your community. The work group will need excellent, easy-to-understand presentation materials, and an organized presentation.

- The governing body considers the elements of a tailored approach for your community, and its members reach consensus. Again, a guided process, using a skilled facilitator with deep understanding of the history to date, is essential. This step will take several meetings at a minimum, and you will likely need to collect additional information from legal or financial consultants during this period.

- Next, the governing body decides how to share the analysis and recommendations with the broader stakeholders and community, including which information to share, and what groups to include.

- A series of discussions is held with the groups identified in the previous step. Consensus-building methods are used, and feedback is solicited and compiled.

- Finally, the governing body reconvenes to incorporate the stakeholder input, and its members reach final consensus on a community model.

You will note that these steps are much more regimented than the previous community processes, because you are moving from an exploratory process into a business planning mode. Don't be surprised if it feels uncomfortable and a bit scary to some or most of the participants. It is!

We suggest you organize your efforts in these steps using the same framework of principal elements that your work group used to study interventions for the uninsured. Here are some tips about choosing an approach for each element.

Principal Element 1 – Care Versus Coverage: Consider whether your underlying issue is access to services, or access to payment for services, and make your case accordingly. There is an important distinction between *coverage* and *insurance*. Insurance products are regulated by individual states, and regulations vary widely. In general, "insurance" involves collecting premiums in exchange for a defined set of benefits, with guarantees to provide those benefits. Under insurance law, federal and state requirements related to minimum benefits and financial reserves must be met.

Medical care coverage that provides dollars for services without charging premiums usually is not subject to such requirements, although there may be other rules that apply in your state. In some states, it is possible to charge premiums for medical care coverage without qualifying as "insurance." In Michigan, the law allows municipalities to provide such coverage. In other states, there are provisions under which the unlicensed subsidiaries of licensed insurers can provide more flexible coverage.

The message here is that the issues of insurance and coverage are different in each state, and are highly complex. We strongly urge you to seek well-informed counsel on this tricky and vitally important issue.

Principal Element 2 – Continuum of Services: Be realistic! There will never be enough resources to meet all your health care needs. Set your sights on objectives that resonate with the community, and address those that you can reasonably achieve. Ignore critics who claim you aren't solving the whole problem. (Neither are they.)

Principal Element 3 – Provider Payment: Understand the historic and current sensitivities in your community, and design strategies with payment levels that the provider community can support. Don't expect certain sectors to carry the burden for others.

Principal Element 4 – Sources of Funding: Our strong bias is for some degree of local funding in every initiative. We believe local funding:

- Builds in strengths of local ownership, investment, and long-term sustainability;

- Keeps people aware of the real burden of health care funding (since it uses your money rather than someone else's);

- Avoids an entitlement basis (which may not be sustained over time); and

- Most effectively integrates local business and social sentiments.

Principal Element 5 – Infrastructure: Let the design of your program drive the infrastructure, and don't shy away from completely re-designing your governance structure if that's what's needed. Remember, form should follow function. Until now, developing a governance model has been a community process; now it must become a business venture.

ACTION TIPS

Step Two Objectives

1. To share an analysis of models from other communities and highlight the elements of successful models that apply to your community's situation.

2. To identify a specific course of action tailored to your community.

3. To generate broad support for your community's selected course of action.

Organizing

We have outlined the organizing steps, in the order we believe they should occur. At this point in your process, you are moving from a community planning process into a more formal business planning process. This calls for a shift in your governance and operations, from models that supported community assessment and planning to models that support program implementation and operation. From this point forward, your governing body and community groups must cooperate with far more detail-oriented issues, reports, and consultants.

It is important to recognize and acknowledge this shift in tone, so that participants are comfortable with it. You will still need community-based leaders and champions who will validate and support the recommendations, but different, more technical experts will be involved in the detailed assessment and design.

Who Pays for This Step?

As in the previous step, you may need resources to employ a skilled facilitator, or you may be fortunate enough to identify someone in your community who has these skills and is willing to donate them to the effort.

Decision Making

At this juncture, it is vital that the governing body make all its decisions by consensus. The committee chair may need to use sophisticated communication strategies to air and address the concerns of each member. There are many consultants and methods available to assist with this process, and you would be wise to engage as much expertise as possible.

Once the governing body agrees on the basic direction of your community's intervention, it is important to engage broader stakeholder input. When presenting the hypothetical model to your community, be open to suggestions for improvement or modification, and bring them back to the governing body. Of course, the governing body retains the final decision-making authority, but it is wise to have incorporated as much community input as possible into those decisions.

Record Keeping

As in previous steps, it is essential to keep an accurate record of decisions. It is also important to keep records of who was invited to participate in the various venues for community input, and who actually participated.

Tips for Conveners

These steps require a great deal of behind-the-scenes work in consensus building, in data gathering, in developing recommendations and presentations, and in managing conflict. To carry them out, it is essential you enlist the services of a skilled facilitator or team of facilitators who have a firm grasp of all of the deliberations to date.

Hazards

- Recall the lessons in Chapter One, and be sure to present all information in terms of its importance to both "camps" of stakeholders — the social and the financial.

- Once again, avoid the temptation to force a hasty end to these steps. Allow time for all community members to think through the analysis and recommendations and to respond with suggestions. Broad-based support of your tailored strategy is absolutely vital. Allow it the time to develop.

- Avoid making the wrong decision because you had inadequate information. Use technical, financial, and legal consultants, and use thorough, analytic business planning methods.

STEP THREE: FORMALIZING THE DETAILED DESIGN OF YOUR MODEL

You have considered a variety of models and determined, with sound rationale, a hybrid model that best suits your community. Now you are ready to move into formalizing the business details and, as they say, "the devil is in the details."

At this juncture, your governing body should formally charge a group with developing an implementation plan for your tailored intervention. This will complete the shift from a community-based process of consensus building to a highly technical process of developing and implementing a business plan. Depending upon your intervention, this process may include some or all of the following elements:

- Actuarial analysis, fee and premium structures;

- Capital outlays;
- Changes in governance or ownership;
- Contracts with providers;

- Contracts with funding sources;
- Data collection methods;
- Financial analysis;
- Facility acquisition or management;
- Identification of outcome and quality indicators;
- Plans for advertising and outreach;
- Regulatory compliance;
- Risk management;
- Sales or enrollment planning; and
- Staffing.

Addressing these issues is far beyond the scope of this manual, and is highly individualized to your situation. But, here is our best advice, based upon our experiences in Muskegon County:

- Recognize that you must address these issues in order to implement a successful program.
- Expect to shift gears into a formal business planning mode at this point.
- Expect to spend money at this point. The financial and legal details are certain to require significant outside consultation, and other issues will, too.
- Expect that these details may take as long as two years to work through.
- Keep communication flowing from your governing body to your community-based teams (who will still be working on their projects) and the community at large throughout the process. Regular updates and status reports, in writing, in the media, and at meetings, will keep interest and momentum peaked.

ACTION TIPS

Step Three Objective

To develop an implementation plan for your community's tailored intervention.

Organizing

The governing body should formally charge a group with developing the implementation plan, completing the shift from a community-based process of consensus building to highly technical business planning. We suggest you structure this step like a technical project, identifying a project manager, subgroups with specialized tasks, an integrated timeline, and formal resource allocation. This will keep efforts focused and organized, and also simplify the reporting to the governing body.

Who Pays for This Step?

This work costs a lot of time and money, and you will need funds. If you secured external funds through a grant or gift earlier, this is where you will use the bulk of the dollars. Depending upon your intervention, there may be local organizations that are willing to contribute resources to this effort. They could include a variety of organizations that are vested in your intervention, such as: health systems; governmental or municipal bodies; community foundations; and employers or corporations.

You also may decide to seek "seed" funds from a foundation or governmental grant programs. *(Note: You need to be thinking about the sources of funds for this work at least six to 12 months before you will need them, because it can take that long to secure them.)*

Decision Making

At some point, depending upon your intervention, formal decision-making may move to an entity other than your governing body. For instance, if you create a new 501(c)(3), the governing body will transfer authority for the intervention to that organization. In other cases, the original governing body may continue.

Tips for Conveners

Regardless of the governance structure, there will be a need to report on progress. Again, we recommend a "project manager" be named and held accountable for reporting to the governance structure. As you proceed into a business plan, facilitation becomes less important and more traditional project progress reporting becomes more important. The governing body's roles are problem solving, acting as public champion, and furnishing oversight for the project.

Hazards

- If you fail to consistently report progress to the community at large, interest will fall away, and momentum and community support will falter.

- Inattention to detail will catch up to you later. You *must* work through all the business details. Use your local business experts as quality control experts if you can — ask them to help you see what you might have missed in legal and financial details, public relations, resource allocation, and other areas.

Chapter.....7

Implementation

- Engaging the Media Effectively
- Managing Politics
- Managing Pent-Up Demand
- Marketing Effectively
- Collecting Data and Reporting Your Progress

In this section, we will bare our souls and share what we wish we had known before we implemented *Access Health©* in Muskegon County. We have learned from our pioneering efforts. We believe that you can learn from them, too, and can use them to implement your local initiative for the uninsured more smoothly and successfully than if we had kept our learning experiences to ourselves.

In retrospect, there are five key areas in which we would change our course if we had the luxury of going back in time. Your early and concerted attention to these issues will save you hardship and heartache. The five key areas are:

- Engaging the media;
- Managing politics;
- Managing pent-up demand;
- Marketing effectively; and
- Collecting data and reporting your progress.

ENGAGING THE MEDIA EFFECTIVELY

Your local media will be an essential partner in your efforts to address the uninsured and under-insured. Just as your community is unique, so is your media.

The number of local newspapers, radio and television stations varies by community, as does the amount of coverage your community receives from surrounding media (e.g., a newspaper published in a nearby larger city). For instance, in Muskegon County, we have just one newspaper and no local radio or television stations. Press from the nearby city of Grand Rapids rarely covers Muskegon. So what shows up in our newspaper is the only thing our residents know about our efforts.

Another variable is the degree to which health care is covered in your local media. The presence of minority, business sector, or other stakeholder media varies, too. What tends *not* to vary is the propensity of the media to take a negative slant, especially in the absence of clearly "good" news.

Our advice is to know your media representatives and to engage them as partners in your efforts to the fullest extent possible. Be careful, and be smart.

From your earliest days, make sure your Steering Committee understands the composition and behavior of your local media. Find out who your media representatives are. Get to know them, and get them involved in your efforts as soon as possible. For instance, local media can serve as a partner in your early efforts to produce a community snapshot by underwriting some of your survey efforts or by adding some of your questions to surveys they already conduct.

Inviting media representatives to serve as members of your Steering Committee may be a possibility, especially if it seems to make political sense. Consider though, that if the media is part of your problem solving apparatus, it must allow the process latitude — negative or premature reporting about your efforts can sabotage your project. If you can't trust your media to give you this latitude (and you will know if you can), don't let them too close to your discovery and decision-making processes.

Several issues fall under the cautionary heading of "be careful." First and foremost, be careful in what you claim you will be able to do for the people in your community.

We made a critical error in Muskegon by declaring our intent to provide coverage to 3,000 people. We made this statement very early in our process, before we understood that it would take several years to reach this goal. Our newspaper seized that number, and in every single article, even positive articles about our success, it points out how we have fallen short of that goal.

In fact, providing coverage for 3,000 people remains our goal and we expect to reach it, although not for a while. But, we can't get our local newspaper to let go of that number and to stop citing us for underachievement. In retrospect, if we had *not* declared our long-term goals in this way, our press coverage would have been far more favorable.

Controlling the timing of the public release of your data, recommendations and interventions is a key tool. Don't rob yourself of that tool by carelessly participating in open meetings.

Be careful of open meeting rules, and recognize that at any meeting governed by these rules, the press has access to any data

Our advice is to know your media representatives and to engage them as partners in your efforts to the fullest extent possible. Be careful, and be smart.

or information you present. Expect full disclosure of everything you bring, and plan accordingly. This means that if your press is hostile to your efforts, or some of your data is time-sensitive, you should keep your preliminary information close to your chest.

Be smart about your own use of the media as a tool. You can reach the public with the message you want them to have by buying media coverage through advertising. If your press or TV/radio stations won't cover you like you want to be covered, use ads and commercials to communicate your message and data the way *you* want them communicated.

We used this strategy very effectively in our community, and you can too. We also crafted press releases about our community "snapshot" as it emerged, so we could control the presentation of this information at our own pace. We have mentioned throughout this manual that timing is very important at many points in the process. Be smart about using your media outlets to support *your* timing.

MANAGING POLITICS

No doubt about it, crafting local interventions for the uninsured and under-insured means changing the manner in which local business is done, a fact that is guaranteed to create local stress. Local stress creates local politics. You will have detractors, non-supporters, and people or groups who want to stop you. We advise you to diligently and consciously plan to address local politics using a two-pronged strategy.

The first prong is to put a few strong, credible personalities right out there in front, to diffuse the power of local negativity (politics) to derail your efforts. Position several of your highly placed, credible Steering Committee members, and later, governing body members, to accept the role of "lightning rod" and to take the heat from highly positioned critics and publicly support your initiative.

The second prong is widespread grassroots support. You will have a number of community-based action teams that are passionately working in their own neighborhoods or within populations you are trying to address. Their many voices supporting your initiative will be a powerful tool in standing down the naysayers. You may need to find places where their voices can be heard, but their testimony is sure to carry weight.

In Muskegon, we believe this two-pronged approach is what saved us from political derailment. But, we believe we "backed into it." We got there by accident, and if we were starting over, we would be much more deliberate in the need for both strategic prongs. We suggest you be more savvy and active than we were in recognizing local politics and addressing them up front.

Another political consideration is Politics, with a capital "P" — engaging your elected officials and your local and state governments. Once you have decided on a direction for your intervention, we urge you to share it with your local officials. Take the time to illustrate how your model works for them and their politics.

We found strong Democratic and Republican support for *Access Health*© because elements of it addressed both their concerns. We also found great value in publicly crediting a variety of local and state legislators for their support during our implementation phase.

MANAGING PENT-UP DEMAND

In creating strategies for the uninsured, we know intuitively that there will be pent-up demand, and that the first people who line up for the new strategy will have a very high level of unmet need and probably active illness.

Since the first people through the door are certain to be high-use clients, and there will not yet be a risk pool containing low-use clients to balance them, you can predict a front-end financial and service drain on your new system. Whether you offer services or coverage, implementation of your model *must* include a strategy for easing into this new business without financially bankrupting it.

You also will need to carefully assess and plan for who your first users will be. In Muskegon, we had several hundred calls about *Access Health*© in the first three days. Gulp. We had to be ready in order to survive.

94

In earlier chapters, we noted the differences between the working and indigent uninsured; there are profound economic implications in those differences. In Muskegon, our per member/per month cost to insure our indigent residents is $64.00, compared with $8.50 for our working uninsured; the service use of these populations differs proportionally. So, if you intend to offer services or coverage to both groups, you may need to "manage" the way the two groups enter your new program.

Variations in pent-up demand also exist within the working uninsured. In Muskegon, we had an unexpected amount of early interest from businesses that were sole proprietors. You'll recall that sole proprietors often have extremely pressing insurance needs, and when they do, it is usually because they are ill. These sole proprietors created a very high financial demand in our program's early days. In retrospect, we should have seen that coming and used a staged strategy to enroll these folks.

Our advice is to predict how the issue of pent-up demand will impact your program, then make the proper service delivery, financing, and enrollment decisions to ensure that you don't fall apart in your first 18 months!

MARKETING EFFECTIVELY

Under the broad heading of marketing, we will address two distinct issues:

- Advertising what you have created to the people who will use it, in terms that will draw them to your service or product (a concept that applies no matter what your intervention is), and
- Selling the product you are offering (which will only apply if, indeed, you are selling a product, like we are).

Advertising your product or service is likely to require more effort and strategy than you assume. No matter what your community intervention, it will only be effective if it reaches the community you wish to serve, and if the individuals in that community hear and respond to it.

It is unlikely that any members of your team will have the professional skills in public relations and advertising that this requires. Even though your public health and safety net providers are probably adept at culturally appropriate outreach, marketing requires additional, specialized skills. We advise you to bring in an experienced marketing professional who can help you at this point.

Having targeted segments of your population for your program, you will need to return to your initial community surveys for clues about where those people go for information about health, who they trust, and what messages both resonate with them and turn them off. Your marketing messages must be built on this information in order to be effective.

For instance, in Muskegon, our target has been the working uninsured. We found that messages like "affordable health care coverage" would actually keep them away from our product. The reason? "Affordable" implies that you have some discretionary revenue with which to buy things. Our target population does not consider that they have discretionary revenue, so "affordable" only means "for someone else." Instead, our advertising campaign uses phrases like "health coverage for about two dollars a day," which is something they can hear and respond to. We never would have known this; it took a marketing professional's perspective.

In returning to our initial community opinion data, we also were reminded that our target population didn't want anything to do with government-sponsored programs. So, we needed to create an advertising strategy that had no entitlement ring to it. Again, a marketing professional was our strength. Your intervention may also need a "brand identity," which is another staple of the marketing profession.

We use a variety of strategies in advertising *Access Health©*. Some of our ads represent the targeted employees in the workplace. Some are targeted specifically at employers, and list the growing number of business participants. Still others show the employer and employee as partners, which is a key feature of *Access Health©*. We also are careful not to mix our ads with information about government-sponsored benefits, because this can be a turn-off for our target audiences.

Marketing strategies need not be expensive, just effective. You need the right message, delivered in the right place at the right time. A *local* marketing consultant will be your best resource. In selecting a marketing consultant, you should look for experience in reaching special populations, as well as a strong knowledge of local marketing opportunities.

Selling a product or service is altogether different. If you are selling something that consumers or business will need to buy, like Muskegon's coverage plan, you will need a sales strategy and qualified sales staff. Like marketing, sales skills are not likely to be a strength of your group. Again, we strongly recommend a consultant. Your sales consultant probably will be someone different from your marketing consultant.

Selling health coverage to a small employer that has not offered it in the past is a tough job. The small employer is difficult to reach. The owner of a day care center, dry cleaner, or small restaurant is working long hours alongside his or her employees. There is little or no "human resource" infrastructure, and these businesses tend not to join Chambers of Commerce. There are very few ways to reach these business owners other than face-to-face. That means someone needs to identify them as potential customers, then get out there, find them, sell them on your product, and sign them up. As you can imagine, this takes time and a competent sales staff.

We should point out that brisk sales are crucial to creating a risk pool that will quickly balance the high-user crowd who sign on first, as discussed previously. In Muskegon, we underestimated the importance of vigorous sales strategies in our early days. If we were starting over, we would build sales strategies into our plan much earlier.

COLLECTING DATA AND REPORTING YOUR PROGRESS

Obviously, if you are providing services or coverage to the uninsured, you will need to collect utilization and cost data. Building these information systems will be part of your pre-implementation activities. What is less obvious is that a sustained, community-driven initiative for the uninsured and under-insured must be evaluated on its *quality* as well.

Client and stakeholder satisfaction are often overlooked, and it is a real challenge to find the resources to collect this information. Also, there is a tendency to ignore client satisfaction in programs for the uninsured. An all-too-common undercurrent among stakeholders is one that says, "These people had nothing without the program, so whatever we give them is better than they had; we can't afford quality."

We urge you to recognize this tendency, and make every effort to move beyond it. To put it simply, if clients don't like the intervention, they won't use it. If they don't use it, their advocates won't like the intervention either, and community support will begin to erode.

Providers and payers need to be surveyed, too, because if they become dissatisfied, community support will erode just as quickly, putting you right back to square one.

This premise goes back to the fundamentals of a community-driven model: you own this intervention, your residents will use it, your providers and payers will be part of it, and you all want it to be good. Your program needs to produce local pride and ownership, and reflect the values and norms of your community. Be prepared to continue to spend time and effort on these important issues, long after your program is launched.

Whatever your initiative, we recommend you design a follow-up survey that will:

- Gauge the public's support of the program;
- Gauge the quality of the service/product delivered, from the *participant's* point of view;
- Gauge the satisfaction with the service/product from the *providers' and payers'* points of view; and
- Study consumers', providers' and payers' reasons for not participating in the initiative.

The type of information you glean from such a survey will allow you to identify the nuances of the population(s) you are serving and refine your products and programs over time. Expect to continue to assess and refine your intervention throughout the course of its lifetime; your willingness to do so and act on your findings will be the key to its longevity.

In Muskegon, we found that young men will not use *Access Health©*. Even though the costs are exceptionally low, they prefer to count on staying healthy, and keep their cash in their pockets.

Epilogue

What **Access Health**[©]
has done for Muskegon County

The efforts that led to *Access Health©* began in Michigan's Muskegon County in 1996 with the formation of a local task force to study our uninsured. We went through all of the steps described in this manual, and, in September 1999, took *Access Health©* to market.

Access Health© is our own program to make health coverage affordable to uninsured working families employed in small to mid-sized businesses in our county. Our typical enrollee is a woman working in the service sector, earning $10.00 per hour or less. Through *Access Health©*, she has coverage for herself and her children for preventive, medical, surgical, and emergency care, but only for services delivered in Muskegon County. More than 200 of our area physicians participate, and more than 300 local businesses have already enrolled in *Access Health©*. An average of 2.6 employees are enrolled per business, and more than 1,500 people have used the program. Also, several hundred children have been identified as eligible for Michigan's Medicaid or SCHP programs.

Since January 2000, more than 300 local businesses have enrolled in *Access Health©* and can now offer local health insurance coverage to their employees and their dependents.

Funding is based on a creative cost-sharing model that fits well with our community's values, norms and politics. Total monthly cost is about $138.00 for single coverage, which is far less than local managed care or traditional insurance options. The employer and employee each pay 30 percent (about $42.00). Providers donate 10 percent of the fees. The remaining 30 percent comes from community match, collected from Disproportionate Share Hospital payments and local government and foundation contributions.

Access Health© has not solved all of Muskegon's uninsured or under-insured problems. But, it has made coverage available to many people who had none; these people can now receive treatment for their asthma, diabetes, high blood pressure, and acute illnesses without bankrupting their families. That makes us proud.

Access Health© has provided a competitive advantage to participating businesses, who can recruit a higher caliber of employee. It has drawn business into our county. It has reduced the burden of uncompensated care for our hospitals and physicians, and has engaged our doctors and health systems as partners with our businesses and safety net providers. That makes us proud, too, and it makes us a stronger community.

We faced many barriers. Often, we were tempted to either fold up and go home or implement an "off-the-rack" solution. Instead, we gutted it out, sometimes running on sheer faith. It was a long three years, but we all agree it was worth it. Our tenacity has paid off. We often remind one another that "amateurs built the Ark, and professionals built the Titanic."

Our homegrown product is tailored to our unique community, and it will serve us for years to come. Because we worked so hard to understand our community and its own unique needs, we are now well prepared to continue to build other customized local efforts.

You can do this, too. And you should. You will find your own strategies to get "Out of the Box and Over the Barriers," and find the right answers for your community. We wish you well.

More Questions? Here's How to Contact Us

If you have further questions about our efforts in Muskegon County, visit our *Access Health©* web site at *www.mchp.org/* or contact us:

Vondie Moore Woodbury
565 W. Western Avenue
Muskegon, MI 49440
Phone 231-728-3201
Fax 231-728-8404
E-mail info@mchp.org

ABOUT THE AUTHORS

Vondie Moore Woodbury directs the Muskegon Community Health Project, which created Access Health©. An politically-savvy community organizer, she has led Muskegon County, Michigan's health improvement efforts for a decade.

Donna Strugar-Fritsch is a consultant in Lansing Michigan, serving a variety of health and human service clients. She has 20 years experience in health care delivery and policy, and has worked with numerous rural communities to develop local health improvement initiatives.

Pamela Paul Shaheen directs the Center for Advancing Community Health in Okemos, Michigan. She has extensive experience in health policy, especially access to health care, and in community change processes.

The authors' combined experiences comprise a complete framework for community-driven health improvement. Recognizing that, they wrote this book.